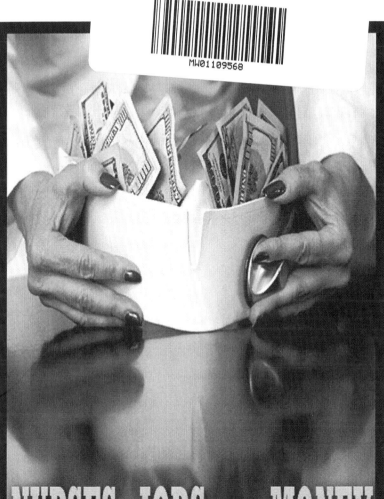

NURSES, JOBS AND MONEY

A Guide to Advancing Your Nursing Career and Salary

CARMEN KOSICEK, RN, MSN

Cover-art-photography: Capture the Canvas Photography: Mikayla Kosicek

Cover graphic designer: Joyce Fler-Reyes

Interior graphic designer: Abul Ala Muhammad Iqbal

Editor: Ocean Cloud Media: Helen Chang

Publishing Company: Visionary LLC

Proudly Printed in the United States of America

First paperback printing: July 2012

ISBN: 0-147-82883-0
ISBN-13: 978-1-4782883-8-1

DEDICATION

This book is dedicated to all my nursing students. Together we have achieved new possibilities for financial and career success, while living our passion as nurses.

CONTENTS

ACKNOWLEDGMENTS

My deepest appreciation goes to my husband, Mike. Without his support and inspiration, this book would not have come to fruition. His encouragement and enthusiasm is instrumental in my success, and I sincerely thank him.

Thanks also to my son, Blake, for helping to streamline many of the technology-driven aspects of this project.

And to my daughter, Mikayla, and her photography business, Capture the Canvas Photography, for the creative cover photo along with the numerous shots for my Facebook page.

Special thanks to the team at Ocean Cloud Media Inc. and editor Helen Chang. Their guidance and direction supported me in progressing smoothly throughout the entire book-writing process.

> "The size of your success is measured by the strength of your desire; the size of your dream; and how you handle disappointment along the way."
>
> — Robert Kiyosaki, *Rich Dad, Poor Dad* and
>
> *The Unfair Advantage*

Chapter 1:
Who's Hiring?

It is well believed that by studying the past, you can "see" the future. Nursing is not any different in this respect. Therefore, it is imperative to begin with looking back, to learn from the past. In my belief, looking back will not only help us to predict the future more reliably, but it will help us to learn where we need to make changes. Really, the root of education is to learn, or to learn from our mistakes, so that the future can be brighter.

Historically, the nursing profession has been dominated by women. True, there are male nurses and even more male nurses as of late, but still, this is a profession predominately made up of women. That being said, let's take a look at the history of women in the workforce and understand how the history is financially impacting us at present.

Maternal work history

Think back for a moment to the time that you were in junior high or high school. Did your mom work? What about your friend's mom? What type of work did your mom or your friend's mom do? Was she climbing the corporate ladder, or was she content with working at a job close to home in the same position for an extended length of time?

My mom worked on her own as a housekeeper when I was in junior high. She worked her hours around the hours of my sisters' and my school and extracurricular schedule. My mom worked very hard so that the money she brought in, extra income for the family, could be used for fun items, in addition to helping with the normal household expenses.

I was in junior high during the mid 80s, and what I just described was common among my friends' mothers at that time. Many women at that time had just re-entered the workforce full time, but many did not have a college degree.

My mom did attend college, but she does not have a college degree. My mom did not work outside the home full time when I was in elementary school. When I was in high school, my mother worked at a company as a secretary full time for a few years. This was typical of my friends' mothers' work histories as well, and it is likely similar to the work histories of women that you know in those age ranges. My dad was the main bread winner, as were my friends' dads. Does that sound like people you know from that generation?

In the 1970s, women began to flood colleges seeking a higher education just like my mother did. Many times these women did not finish college, or if they did, they did not have intentions of working full time and utilizing the education as the main bread winner of the family.

However, women of that generation who completed college gained the choice to work or not, and this opportunity was a drastic change from what their mothers experienced in relation to working outside the home. That is to say, my grandmother's generation did not typically seek higher education and were not expected to be employed full time outside the home. Additionally, if women of my mother's generation did go to college, they typically studied education or nursing.

First generation

Why is this important? This historical overview directly relates to women's earning potential in today's current age.

"How?" you may ask. You see, *we* are the first generation of women who are planning to have long-term gainful employment as one of the integral members--or in some cases, as the main bread winner--of the family.

Why do we care about this historical pattern? Because more likely than not, the nurse manager that you are seeking gainful employment from is from my mother's generation. The nurse manager from whom you are trying to get a job interview—and consequently a job—looks at you and subconsciously thinks back to her/his past and reflects upon the historical pattern of working women.

The majority of women in my mother's generation did work before they got married. However, they often did not work full time while their children were young. The women in the previous generation who did work were more likely to leave the workforce to have children or would work part time when raising their children.

These patterns of the past affect today's hiring habits, and may jeopardize employers' decisions regarding job promotions. For example, an employer may unconsciously or subconsciously reflect on the historical working patterns of women. Thus, with the case of the female worker, the employer may subconsciously feel that the worker might leave her job at any time to return to the job of raising the family.

Ultimately, this can lead to less opportunity for advancement. Additionally, most prestigious positions have historically been held by men, and again, a subconscious reflection on this matter may keep women out of the highest-paid positions, simply due to the preconceived working pattern of women.

Sadly, this pattern often continues, since the network of people in those prestigious positions often lead to hiring others who are similar to them. Thus, the working pattern is perpetuated, and women continue to be underrepresented in the best jobs.

Working patterns

Fast forward to your generation. More than likely, *you* are planning to work full time even while your children are young. In today's times, it often takes more than one income to make ends meet. Perhaps you chose to work full time to save for the future because you will not have an employer-sponsored full pension to rely on in retirement. Or perhaps you chose to work full time, because you are single and do not plan on marrying. Or you may be a single parent. Whatever the reason, more women are working full time than in past generations.

Pay gaps

As if this wasn't enough, it is important to understand that despite current equal pay laws, women historically earn less than men for the same role, even when a woman and a man have the same experience and educational background.

One of the factors behind this pay gap may be that the nurse manager who is from my mother's generation may subconsciously think to her past when she analyzes resumes before she even considers requesting an interview with a particular candidate. When a male candidate is selected for an interview, the nurse manager may subconsciously think that the male is the main bread winner or perhaps that the male is more likely to keep employment full time over a longer period of time. Historically speaking, it is more likely that a male nurse in the past would also have had a higher college degree than his female counterpart, since it was not until the 70s that the volume of women flooded the collegiate system.

So now let's pretend that *you* are a hiring nurse manager. A woman and a man of equal educational and experiential background are presented to you. It is your decision which to hire. Again, if all things are equal, do you see why the men are potentially in a highly sought after position?

Furthermore, if you are a nurse manager in today's economy, how do you entice a male nurse to accept the position that you need to fill? More likely than not, with higher pay, of course!

It isn't as if the nurse manager can offer more vacation time or a higher-matching percentage to the 401(k) plan to her staff nurse. Think about it. What the nurse manager *can* offer is higher pay.

You see, this is a large part of why male nurses make more than their female counterparts, even if their experience and education levels are equal.

> "For your own good, for the good of your family and your future, grow a backbone. When something is wrong, stand up and say it is wrong, and don't back down."
>
> — Dave Ramsey, *The Total Money Makeover: A Proven Plan for Financial Fitness*

The nurse next to you

Let's think about the following scenario. In a hospital setting, registered nurses (RNs) in a particular hospital unit basically have the same job status and pay range, no matter what their clinical experience or educational background is.

For example, if you walk into the obstetrics (OB) unit of a hospital, all the labor and delivery (L&D) RNs -- no matter what their education or experience levels are -- basically have the same job status. They are all considered staff RNs who work in L&D.

One staff RN could have an associate degree or bachelor's degree in nursing, while the one right next to her could be an RN with a Master of Science in Nursing (MSN). Yet, they both function as staff RNs, and their pay is similar. In addition, these RNs have a general idea as to what the other RNs are making.

You would not think that one staff nurse for the same employer, say Hospital ABC, would be paid $65.00 an hour while another staff RN in the same unit is making $30.00 an hour (not taking into account call pay/overtime/shift differential/etc.), but generally the base pay would be similar within a range.

Equal is not equal

This matters, because when the women compare their income to other women, they realize they are in the same pay range and thus conclude that their pay is fair. Since the nursing field has predominately been dominated by women, the women are then satisfied, because they are comparing their pay against other women.

Nowadays, more men are becoming nurses and they are being paid at a higher level. To me, this is not satisfying. To me, when this information is unearthed about the inequality in pay, it should not simply be swiped under the rug.

It is not the male nurses' fault. Rather, it is the fault of the women and men who allow this cycle of inequality in pay to continue by being silent. Also, a majority of women who learn about the inequality of pay are less assertive and less confrontational than men regarding the matter, and they are less willing to ask for a pay raise to equal the playing field. These are yet additional contributing factors that often lead to inequalities in pay, since larger raises often go to the *men* who aggressively ask for them!

For me, this totally frosts my cake. I have worked *very* hard to obtain a graduate degree in nursing, along with multiple graduate certificates. However, should I settle on making 20-percent less than men on average, simply because I am not male?

National statistics from varying employment articles show that a woman makes 80 cents of every $1.00 that a man makes – and this is in 2012! It is time for a change.

Women Make Less Than Men

"In 1963, when the Equal Pay Act was signed, women made 59 cents on average for every dollar earned by men (based on Census figures of median wages of full-time, year-round workers). By 2009, women earned 77 cents to men's dollar, a narrowing of the wage gap by less than half a cent a year. Over a working lifetime, this wage disparity costs the average American woman and her family an estimated $700,000 to $2 million, impacting Social Security benefits and pensions."

- The National Committee on Pay Equity (www.pay-equity.org/)

The good news

I can show you a different way to approach your nursing career and obtain the pay and recognition that you deserve. If you learn how to increase your pay early on in your nursing career, can you imagine the positive changes that *you will be able to bring to your* family?

Cycle of unequal pay

It is high time that nurses and women teach other women and men how to level the playing field. Also, it is imperative that male nurses learn this historical pattern as well. *Why*? Because most likely, it will be the men in nursing that are promoted to the higher positions. Thus, it is likely that in the future, the men that are in the higher nursing positions will be doing the hiring of future nurses.

If nurses are not educated now about the historical disparity in pay and the potential subconscious reasoning behind that disparity, then the cycle of unequal pay will continue in the years to come. Again, this is because men and women in hiring positions may have a tendency to look subconsciously to their past when making decisions about whom to hire and how much to pay him or her.

Breaking the cycle

People react to what they believe is true. This past working pattern *was* true, but now a new truth has emerged. And once the old truth is completely exposed, the new truth can be made transparent. It can be openly communicated amongst a profession of educated people, thus ending the cycle of unequal pay.

I am excited to share with you secrets I have learned in nursing, business and healthcare economics. But the bigger question is: Once you learn my knowledge, will you choose to merely hold on to the information, or will you choose to implement what you have learned and increase your earning potential? Ask yourself,

"Will I be up to the challenge? Will I become successful? Will I be as good as or better than those who came before me?"

In order to succeed, you must build your *knowledge*, take *action* and overcome your *fear*. I will tell you this over and over again throughout this book. You must take the knowledge that I have given you – about historical female working patterns, misconceived notions about today's female working patterns and inequalities in pay due to gender – and combine that with action to break the vicious cycle and clear the path for today's generation of nurses.

Chapter 2:

Get a Job While in School

Perhaps you are still in nursing school, and wondering how you will land a job, because you do not yet have any experience in the healthcare field. Or perhaps you have not worked outside the home in a while. The great news for you is that you are reading this *now,* and I can give you some ideas to help you not only in your job search but in successfully landing a position!

Many times, I see newly graduated nurses who are frustrated with hearing that although they now have the right education, they still cannot land a hospital nursing position because they do not have any experience.

Quite frankly, education is not enough in today's nursing job market. *Experience* is the key. This is because, in school, exposure to the nursing world is accomplished via clinical rotations. However, depending on the nursing program (an associate-degree nursing program may not spend the same amount of time on clinical rotations as a bachelor's-degree nursing program), this exposure process varies. Unfortunately, what is constant is that in every situation the clinical hours and clinical experiences that the nursing student is exposed to are limited.

Once you have graduated from your nursing program, you must realize that a hospital's primary reason for not hiring too many newly graduated nurses is mainly one of safety. Each hospital unit can only have a certain percentage of nursing staff that has little experience. So, how do you gain experience if no one will help you to get the experience? Well, there is a technique for that! And yes, I will show you what it is!

Create your experience

Let me now share an example that is outside the realm of nursing, since often the forest cannot be seen from the trees. I know of a young lady who was interested in photography. However, no one would give her a job as a photographer, since she was a young teenager at the time. No matter how strong her passion or desire or willingness to work was, her lack of experience was stopping her in her tracks.

I suggested to her that she call a photographer and help him or her out for free. Novel idea! Not really, but it is one that is not used as often as it could be! Anyway, this young lady purchased a newspaper, looked at the by-line beneath the photographs to find out who the photographer was and started calling them up the "old-fashioned" way, person to person. With enthusiasm she let the photographers know that she had great news to share with them. Of course, they listened. Who would *not* want to know great news, after all?

She went on to inform them that she was working on a project that would afford them *free* help at photo shoots. She would be there to assist them with carrying around equipment, running professional errands, etc. Then, she went on to ask if they would be interested in a few hours of her free time. *Two* photographers–of the small handful that she called—accepted the free help! She had just landed her first two internships, which now put her in a leveraged position. These would give her needed experience.

Experience on paper and in life is about what you make of opportunity. This young lady did go and help with carrying equipment. … And she brought along her camera and took shots as well. Additionally, she had the photographers give her input on her images, and they requested that she return to take more photos.

After six intensive internships, this young lady could list her experience with well-known photographers in the area, and she started to work on her own. The photographers have since aided her with building a network within the photography community as well.

Now, this young lady has a *thriving* private photography business at the whopping age of nearly 17. To this day, she still interns with photographers since she understands that the internships lead to more networking opportunities and more experience.

Internships

If this is your situation, I would highly suggest an internship! An internship is typically geared for professional careers and where you can gain supervised practical experience. For the supervising professional, there is usually no cost to hire the intern and it creates a sense of professional and personal pride in enhancing the knowledge of an intern. For the intern, the benefits are gainful experience in a particular field and making contacts within that professional area of study.

What, you do not know how to create your own internship? Well then, let me help you! First of all, it is imperative to point out that the internship that I am suggesting is *not* being done for classroom credit and you are *not* going to go through your school, college or university to set this up. Again, your school, college or university is not creating the internship; you are.

Since your school, college or university is not the one paying your school loans, but you are, then *you* are the one who needs to take accountability for making your future happen. When you actually think about it, an internship is a *volunteer* activity after all, so how can a school, college or university stop you from volunteering for an activity that is not associated with the learning institution? Besides, you are advancing your education and wouldn't the school agree that they want you to learn both outside *and* inside the classroom?

Again, remember that this internship is not associated with your learning institution! So keep in mind that since it is not associated with your institution, you will *not* have the school, college or university's malpractice insurance to cover you. Also, you cannot wear a school uniform or name tag that is associated with your learning institution while volunteering at your internship.

> **"When you are young, work to learn, not to earn."**
>
> — Robert Kiyosaki, *Rich Dad, Poor Dad* and *The Unfair Advantage*

Learn to earn

You are young in your nursing career, and since you are still in school, *now* is the time to work for free so that you can learn. Remember, you can be *young* at something in your career at any age. For example, if you have been a staff nurse for 20 years and you now want to do something different, such as become a nurse navigator, nurse risk manager, legal nurse consultant, nurse liaison, nurse educator, etc., you are young in that desired portion of your career. If this describes your current situation, I would highly suggest that you create and participate in an internship!

Remember, statistically speaking, there is only a small percentage of the population who have participated in an internship. So just imagine how impactful this will be perceived on your resume under the heading of "experience"! Additionally, hospitals simply want to hire nurses who have more clinical time under their belts... And now you will stand out in a crowd of applicants because you *will* have more time in a hands-on setting!

Create your internship

So, *how* do you create your own internship? First you need to know that to be in most nursing programs, you need to have some sort of medical insurance that covers yourself for certain healthcare needs. So, make an appointment with your medical provider, using your medical insurance. That is right, schedule an appointment with your OB/GYN or your primary care physician (PCP), whether it is an internal medicine or family practice physician, or schedule an appointment with your child's pediatrician! Preferably, you will be able to make an appointment with a medical provider that you know, but this does not have to be the case. It will simply increase your odds of creating an internship with that person.

Next, go to the scheduled appointment. By this point, you may realize that you are not going to use your appointment to ask for medical advice or treatment from the chosen medical provider. What you really made this appointment for is to have a scheduled time during which you can talk to the provider about the unpaid internship that you would like to create and participate in! Additionally, you are paying the provider to speak with him or her, so he or she must listen to you! Genius!

What to say

Once you have the medical provider's attention, look at the provider and say, "I have great news for you!" He or she will be excited, because you have just told the person that you have something that will help him or her in some way. Do you see how this opening is already better than asking the medical provider to help you, which can cause the provider to either react defensively or tune you out completely?

Next, tell the provider, "I have free help for your office!" Seriously, even if he or she is not a self-employed provider, how could the person not want something for *free*?

Then go on to remind the provider what Hillary Clinton told every American several years back: "It takes a village!" Then remind the person about what he or she went through in medical school and that everyone needs a bit of help to succeed in this industry.

Now go ahead and say to the provider, "I need an internship."

Time for an internship

Most internships last 12 weeks. You are probably wondering how you are going to fit this into your already hectic schedule. Stop it. I did not say that you will have to volunteer for 40 hours a week for 12 weeks, but you will have to put in some time. You also need to think about this from the perspective of your future resume, which is severely lacking any kind of health care experience.

On your resume, your options are to write that "I worked at hospital XYZ for 12,800 hours" or that "I worked at hospital XYZ from July of 2012 to November of 2012." Clearly, it is most accepted as the norm to write your time in the number of months and years, not hours. So when you list your internship experience on your resume, you are going to describe it as lasting for three months. I do not care how many hours you volunteer per week at the internship for those three months – and neither will your prospective employer. Remember that either way you are *ahead* of the vast majority of applicants because you have had a one-on-one internship. Thus, you have increased your hours, in contrast to the other nursing applicants who only have clinical hours from their school programs.

Present this internship idea with all these details to your medical provider. Again, it does not matter what type of medical provider you approach, because that provider has friends in all areas of the hospital! That provider knows nurse managers, the ones who eventually have shortages in their units. You are building a *network* here!

Benefits to the medical provider

Once your provider says "yes" to your proposal, you need to talk to the office nurse. It is a strong possibility that the office nurse does not have a graduate degree and therefore does not think that she or he is qualified to teach. But you have great news for this person! Now, the office nurse can engage in a teaching role with *you,* and she or he can add "instructor" to her or his resume! This is a win-win situation!

To point out the benefit of your internship to the office nurse, you can say, "I have great news for you! Doctor So-and-So is bringing me in for an internship. Since I will be working with you as well, *you* can legitimately add the title of 'instructor/teacher' to your resume! After all, I will be learning a great deal from you." More than likely, the office nurse will be pleased to be able to add another title to her or his resume.

When your internship starts, jump right in and help, ask questions. Just think, since *you* created this role, you will not have to submit school clinical papers such as care plans or logs, as you would in a school-related clinical rotation. So instead, contribute a lot in a clinical sense! Unlike a clinical rotation, the internship "students" *desire* to be present! After all, this, unlike the clinical rotation, is not a mandate or a school requirement. Internships highlight the students who *want* to be present to learn!

No connections

"Deidra" was a student nurse seeking a bachelor's degree and had only been in the United States for a few years. She previously worked at a large industrial manufacturing company, but lacked experience in healthcare, or in customer service for that matter.

She had a young, school-aged son, but none of her family lived near her, so she lacked connections.

When I spoke of my internship technique one day in class, Deidra lit up. She feverishly took notes on what to say, and at the clinical rotation, she and I rehearsed. A few weeks passed, and Deidra excitedly called to say that she had landed an internship. It happened during an appointment with her son's pediatrician. She had asked him – in the same fashion that she had rehearsed with me – about creating an internship for her. The MD, who worked as an employed physician of a large healthcare system, said that he would go through the proper channels to see if Deidra could be the first intern in that office. Deidra was on cloud nine! She was so excited to know that the MD had listened to her and considered her request.

A few weeks later, Deidra came up to me at class and hugged me. The MD had said yes to her internship! Deidra knew now that, not only did the technique work, but that she was taking positive, proactive steps to build her resume, which in turn increased the likelihood of her landing a position upon graduation.

Make your resume pop

"Monique," an associate-degree-seeking student nurse of mine, recently learned this same technique. Monique is a married mother of four children, who lives in a rural town and has not been part of the paid workforce outside of the home for many years. Monique is a *perfect* candidate for an internship.

Do you see why? Remember, this is not only a resume-building technique, but a networking opportunity! Monique stands to dually benefit from this technique.

When you highlight your internship on your resume, it will *make your resume pop*!

Also, nowadays, many people have lost the wisdom of why it is so extremely valuable to work for free when they are young – and again, I don't merely speak of one's age. I mean that it's valuable to work for free while you are young in your career!

Increase your chances

Here are some other insights to consider with your internship. Your medical provider may or may not realize that in some parts of the country, RN positions are challenging to come by. After you have completed your first internship, you can network with the provider to help create another internship with another provider. The first provider may also be able to help you network with providers who are hiring and help you better position yourself for your first RN position! Nothing is a guarantee, but these techniques can increase your chances of landing that RN job after you graduate or even increase your chances of landing a student nurse position while you are in school!

The importance of a degree

Are you currently in school for an associate degree of science in nursing and want to save *thousands* of dollars on your following bachelor's degree of science in nursing?

If an associate degree is your only degree thus far, it is *highly* recommended that you continue on for a bachelor's degree in nursing. Seriously, do not stop your schooling in nursing if you only have an associate degree. Highlighting the importance of a BSN degree is the Institute of Medicine, IOM's, national campaign for action, which began in November 2010. One of the recommendations of the IOM is to increase the proportion of nurses with a baccalaureate degree to 80 percent by the year 2020 (http://thefutureofnursing.org/recommendations).

I know that right now this may be gut-wrenching to even think about, but I really am about to save you thousands of dollars if you are already at a zero estimated family contribution, EFC, on your Free Application for Federal Student Aid, FAFSA.

False hope

The majority of you falsely believe that your future employer will fully fund your schooling for a bachelor's degree. But, go ahead, take a moment right now, look up a variety of employers online and find information about their education-funding programs. I bet that a majority of those employers will simply fund $5,000 or *less per year* in educational expenses that directly relates to your employment *if* you pass the course – and if you work full time.

Also, if you do not have a bachelor's degree, the RN to BSN completion programs, which take 18 months or more to complete online, run around $10,000 - $20,000 or more. Clearly, your employer will not come close to paying 100 percent of that cost in the approximately 18-month timeframe! If, however, someone had a chat with you *now*, you could decrease the amount of money you spend on obtaining your BSN – by a significant amount – as well as increase your odds of gaining employment as a RN!

Spend less on school

Here we go! Take notes!

For the following scenario that we will run, let's assume that our subject is an independent student as defined by the federal government. Make sure you follow the federal government's rules and guidelines regarding how to properly designate student status!

The following is from an article regarding "Dependent vs. Independent" status for students from Fastweb.com.

"In the federal government's eyes, all students are considered primarily responsible for funding their higher education. But the government also recognizes that most parents contribute financially on some level. Parents provide assistance whether they've been saving for years to fund their child's degree or simply provide housing while their children study.

"Taking this into account, the federal government applies two different standards for students, one for dependent students and one for independent students. Dependent students are assumed to have parental support while independent students are not. The result: Independent students might qualify for more aid.

"Being considered an independent student is not merely a matter of being responsible for your own educational expenses. You must meet at least one of the following seven criteria to be declared an independent student for the purposes of the FAFSA:

    Be 24 years of age or older by December 31 of the ward year;

    Be an orphan (both parents deceased), ward of the court, or was a ward of the court until the age of 18;

    Be a veteran of the Armed Forces of the United States;

    Be a graduate or professional student;

    Be a married individual;

Have legal dependents other than a spouse;
Be a student for whom a financial aid administrator makes a documented determination of independence by reason of other unusual circumstances."

Changing your status – Dependent students may change their status, but it's not easy. You start by filing a Dependency Review Form; request one from your school. You also must provide documentation explaining your situation. Your case is then reviewed by a committee or financial aid office at your college.

"Keep in mind that most students will not qualify for a change in status. Circumstances tend to be extreme (such as abandonment or physical abuse) to warrant the change. Simply residing in your own apartment or house is not adequate justification.

"If you think you have unusual circumstances that would qualify you as an independent, speak with a financial aid administrator at your school."

Government awards

The amount of money that the federal government will give you for student aid or FAFSA (Free Application for Federal Student Aid) is determined by the amount of income, assets and student dependency status. Keep in mind that income taxes are figured one year in the rears. So, to maximize the amount that you are awarded, you should apply for *FAFSA money* when your income is the lowest, meaning when you are a student, especially an independent, low-asset-low-income student!

Loosely speaking, if your taxable income is $50,000 or less and your assets are in an acceptable range (to find out if your assets are in an acceptable range, visit FinAid.org), your Estimated

Family Contribution or EFC (i.e., how much you and your family will need to contribute toward your school costs), will be low. In turn, your FAFSA award will be greater. Clearly, an EFC of zero is the lowest out-of-pocket expense, but that does not necessarily mean that you do not pay anything out of pocket for college.

For more information, try going to Google and searching "EFC Calculators." Then run a few scenarios that pertain to your specific situation. For instance, if your EFC is high, look up articles on how to "lower my EFC." Remember that these guidelines are based on tax laws, so you should consult a certified public accountant or CPA who specializes in college planning.

If you are an independent-status student with a low EFC, I highly recommend that you start your BSN completion *right now* if you have not done so already. If you piggyback your BSN directly onto your associate degree in nursing (ADN) – meaning that you complete the two degrees back to back – you will maximize as much FAFSA money as possible, and you can apply for tuition reimbursement with your new employer if it is offered! Yeah! Oh, also, applying to a Magnet-Status or Magnet-Seeking-Status Organization as a BSN-enrolled RN is *huge* if you apply!

Magnet status

Time out. What exactly does "Magnet status" mean? Magnet status describes a healthcare organization that has been granted a specific award title, granted by the American Nurses' Credentialing Center or ANCC (which is an affiliate of the American Nurses Association or ANA), for quality patient care, nursing excellence and innovations in professional nursing practice.

The Magnet status recognition award is viewed as the ultimate credential for a healthcare organization that has high-quality, successful nursing practices and strategies -- which in turn deliver excellent patient outcomes – while having high levels of nursing job satisfaction, low nursing staff turnover and pertinent grievance resolution. The Magnet status is fast becoming a worldwide phenomenon.

The term arose from a study of 163 hospitals in the early 1980s that helped to chronicle specific traits that promote an environment within healthcare organizations that not only attracts but retains well-qualified nurses, who in turn promote quality patient care. Of the 163 healthcare organizations studied, 41 exemplified traits that drew in and retained quality nurses, and therefore had outstanding outcomes. Thus, the term "magnet" arose to describe the 41 outstanding organizations.

Ideally, Magnet-status organizations involve nurses not only in data collection, but in the decision-making processes within the patient care delivery model. For instance, "The goal of Magnet nursing leaders is to value staff nurses and have an inclusive environment forming research-based nursing practice, and encourage and reward them for advancing in nursing practice. Magnet hospitals are supposed to have open communication between nurses and other members of the health care team, and an appropriate personnel mix to attain the best patient outcomes and staff work environment."

I point out this information about the Magnet award because it emphasizes the importance of having a bachelor's degree in nursing. For example, any nurse that wants to apply for Magnet status or to work at a Magnet-status hospital is encouraged to have at least a bachelor's degree. This is insightful since a lot of experienced nursing staff members do not have bachelor's degrees. Staff RNs do not need to have a bachelor's degree; although, again, Magnet-status nurses are highly encouraged to do so. Thus, having a bachelor's degree is important for any nurse who wants to stand out from the rest of the competition.

AD vs. BS degrees

I have been a nursing instructor at both bachelor-degree-seeking nursing programs and at associate-degree-seeking nursing programs. Personally, I do not see much difference between the nursing curriculums that are taught at either of these programs. However, I do agree that RNs should have a bachelor's degree simply because it promotes professionalism, creates a standard baseline and increases the breadth of knowledge that a professional is exposed to, given the varied and numerous courses that this person was exposed to as a student.

Let me share an example outside of nursing. Would you be comfortable with a teacher, an accountant or an engineer who does not have a bachelor's degree as a minimum requirement? I would not. Although many people are fabulous at what they do because they have amassed many years of professional experience – even though they do not have a bachelor's degree – they do not have a wide base of knowledge that is recognized as the collegiate standard within academia. Also, those without a bachelor's degree may not have a wide base of experience with working with various institutions. Sadly, these people are often the ones who are left unprepared when they are downsized.

Stability myths

No job is completely stable, especially in our current economy. So, to debunk the myth that nursing is a stable profession, may I remind you of what people used to think about automotive-industry jobs, banking-industry jobs or perhaps federal postal-system jobs? You are smirking, right? Then *why* do you think that healthcare industry jobs, such as nursing jobs, are any different? Why do you think that nursing jobs are bullet proof? *They are not.* When economic conditions are difficult – as in today's times – even more jobs are at risk.

New truths

Why do you still hold on to old beliefs when the truth is staring you in the face right now? What else have I already shown you that you are choosing not to see or believe? In case you still doubt what I say, think about the following examples that I have pulled straight from news headlines throughout the United States. These headlines highlight the fact that within the medical industry, financial weakness is showing up more and more nationally.

- As of the spring 2012, skilled nursing facilities nationwide plan on cutting nursing positions as well as freezing new hire positions, due to the federal financial cuts in Medicare and Medicaid. Sadly, 36.8 percent of facilities surveyed nationally plan to reduce staff, according to The Alliance for Quality Nursing Home Care.

- In April 2012, one of the major Florida city newspapers featured a hospital system where more than 369 full-time nurses were being eliminated and replaced with part-time nursing staff.

- In March 2012, *The New York Times* ran a story stating that 240 nurses, doctors and other workers were laid off from a local New York hospital.

- In a northern suburb of Chicago in March 2012, a hospital laid off 104 employees due to their reported $13.2 million operational loss in 2011, according to a *Crain's Chicago Business* report. This lay-off accounted for 3 percent of the hospital's work force.

Prepare for your career

I am not trying to convey an attitude of doom and gloom, but rather, I am showing you why you *need* to prepare. You *need* to build your base of knowledge and experience – and build it strong and wide – because you will need it. It is better to build it now when you do not need it so that when you inevitably do need it, you will have it. Ask yourself, "Do you want to be ahead of the trend or behind it?"

> **"Walk away from the 97 percent crowd. Don't use their excuses. Take charge of your own life."**
>
> -- Jim Rohn

If you do not already have a bachelor's degree, I highly recommend that you go on for a bachelor of science degree in nursing, BSN. Why? Look back at the Magnet-status discussion, and that alone should make the future path of nursing quite clear as to what will be needed to set you apart from the competition.

Your BSN

If you are an independent student whose income, assets and EFC are low, *why* would you wait to complete your BSN until you are working full time? You see, once you start working, your income will have increased and you may not qualify for the low EFC. Then you will be *stuck* paying for most of your college costs with *only* tuition reimbursement from your employer to help compensate.

If you qualify *now* for a low EFC, then right now is the time to sign up to start on your BSN education! *Do not* wait even one semester! Jump in right now to maximize the financial help that is available to you for college. I know, it may be gut wrenching to think about going on for more schooling, but if you are going to end up going on anyway, why not maximize the financial help that is available to you now?

Just in case my previous message was not direct enough, let me reiterate that if you do not already have a bachelor's degree and you are in an associate degree program for nursing, you should *apply now* for your RN-BSN bridge program. That means, get going!

For FAFSA reasons, you need to apply for your BSN program *now* if you only have one or two semesters left of your associate degree nursing program or ADN. Do not wait until you have completed your ADN! Remember, being admitted into a BSN program can take more than a semester, and the time is ticking with FAFSA.

Choose the money college

Believe it or not, the most important equation for all this strategic college financial planning has been around for quite some time, and I bet that most of you do not even know it exists. It is

<u>COA-EFC=(NEED/HGP)+(SD)=TC</u>. This formula was created by our elected representatives in Washington, DC and was amended by the Obama administration.

Here is a list of definitions from <u>azcollegeplanning.com</u> to help you understand this important formula:

- <u>COA</u> is the Total Cost of Attendance for one full year. This includes tuition, labs, books, room & board, travel, other expenses and fees.

- The <u>EFC</u> is the federal formula for creating your "out of pocket portion" of college expenses. This is the cost that you are required to pay before you get any financial aid. This is what we have focused our discussion around.

- <u>NEED</u> is calculated by subtracting the EFC from the COA.

- <u>HGP</u> is the Historical Giving Pattern. This number is reported to the Department of Education. This is the average amount of financial aid given. In other words, it is how much, historically speaking, a particular college/university has given away in free money. Remember, this amount can change, but it reflects the historical trends of that college/university.

- <u>SD</u> is the student desirability. A college or university may desire one student over another for a variety of reasons and is thus apt to hand out financial aid to attract certain types of students. This can be especially true if the students have already proven themselves with college-level courses.

- **TC** is the True Cost. In other words, this is how much it will really take to go to a particular college or university for one year.

Given this information, which college should you choose to continue at? Well, personally, I would research each college or university to find out how much free money the institution gives away. That is right, *free money*! Go to CollegeBoard.org to look up any college in the search bar on the left; then click on the "paying" tab, and it will tell you the historical giving pattern, HGP, of that college — meaning, in general, how much money that college *gives away for free*! You can go onto the CollegeBoard.org website and look for the percentage of money that the college gives away in scholarships, as in free money! Nope, I am not kidding.

Should you need further help with this, do not hesitate to visit our website NursingCareerProfessionals.com and reach out to us.

I will show you how this all comes together as we next financially examine two different colleges from the CollegeBoard.org site. Please note that this example was calculated off of the 7/2012 information found on CollegeBoard.org .

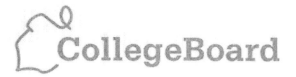

Compare two colleges

COLLEGE #1: **Northern Illinois University in DeKalb, Ill.**

Follow along with our examples by visiting CollegeBoard.org. In the search bar that is on the left-hand side of the landing page, type in "Northern Illinois University." Under the "Paying" tab, you should see this:

Northern Illinois University
DeKalb, IL
Published Annual College Costs Before Financial Aid
(Fall 2011 First Year Students)

In-State Costs			
	On Campus	Off Campus	At Home
Tuition and fees	$11,484	$11,484	$11,484
Room and board	$10,648	--	--
Books and supplies	$1,400	$1,400	$1,400
Estimated personal expenses	$2,396	--	--
Transportation expenses	$700	--	--
Estimated Total	**$26,628**	**$12,884**	**$12,884**

Financial Aid Distribution

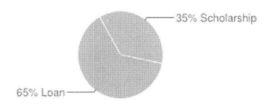

Undergraduate aid typically awarded as shown

65%
% of need met

85%
% of freshmen with financial aid

Calculate Your Net Price / True Cost (TC)

Financial aid can include grants, loans, scholarships and work-study jobs. Every student's financial aid package varies depending on individual circumstances. This is where the HGP (Historical Giving Pattern) comes into play.

Look at the estimated total cost per year for an in-state student who lives on campus, the COA (Total Cost of Attendance) is $26,628. Of that amount, 65 percent of the total cost need is met, which means that the COA, $26,628 x .65 (the percentage of need met) = $17,308, is taken care of upfront in either scholarships/grants/loans. But to even attend, *you* need to come to the table with $9,320 ($26,628 - $17,308 = $9,320).

How much does this university give away in *free* money? Look at the pie graph where it show how much is available in scholarships. They give away 35 percent -- 35%, of the $17,308. That means that $6,057 ($17,308 x .35 = $6,057) is available free, and the rest, $11,250 ($17,308 x .65 –pie graph shows 65% in loan is available = $11,250), is available to you in the form of a loan and the $9,320, remember, you need to come up with on your own.

So, the total out-of-pocket expense for this school is the initial unmet amount of $9,320 plus the loan amount of $11,250, which equals a total amount of $20,570 – *if* you meet the FAFSA zero EFC and other guidelines and *if* you are awarded all of the available scholarships at the maximum amount.

Keep in mind that this example is just to give you a well-guesstimated ballpark idea of college costs and financial aid distribution. I know, I know, in my example, I figured the total expenses based on the reported on-campus-living expenses, but remember, this is just a demonstration so that you can learn how to run your own numbers. If you had no clue as to how these financial aid awards letters were calculated, now you do!

Lastly, keep in mind that, when you call the college to inquire about scholarships, they will tell you, more often than not, that scholarships are need and/or merit based. "Need" is determined by your taxes as discussed above, and FAFSA will determine that for you. A zero EFC shows that you need the most free money. "Merit" is driven by your GPA.

COLLEGE #2: **Trinity College in Hartford, Conn.**

Follow along with our examples by visiting CollegeBoard.org. In the search bar that is on the left-hand side of the landing page, type in "Trinity College." Under the "Paying" tab, you should see this:

Trinity College
Hartford, CT
Published Annual College Costs Before Financial Aid
(Fall 2011 First Year Students)

In-State Costs			
	On Campus	Off Campus	At Home
Tuition and fees	$45,730	$45,730	$45,730
Room and board	$11,800	$11,800	$4,140
Books and supplies	$1,000	$1,000	$1,000
Estimated personal expenses	$1,000	$900	$900
Transportation expenses	$250	$250	$250
Estimated Total	**$59,780**	**$59,680**	**$52,020**

Financial Aid Distribution

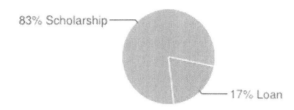

83% Scholarship

17% Loan

Undergraduate aid typically awarded as shown

100%
% of need met

86%
% of freshmen with financial aid

Calculate Your Net Price/ True Cost (TC)

Financial aid can include grants, loans, scholarships and work-study jobs. Every student's financial aid package varies depending on individual circumstances. This is where the HGP (Historical Giving Pattern) comes into play.

Look at the estimated total cost per year for an in-state student who lives on campus, the COA (Total Cost of Attendance) is $59,780. Of that amount, 100 percent of the need is met, which means that of the total price to attend, $59,780 or 100 percent of that, is taken care of upfront in either scholarships/grants/loans. So, to even attend, *you* do not need to come to the table with anything!

How much does this college give away in *free* money? Look at the pie graph where it show how much is available in scholarships.

They give away 83 percent – 83%, of $59,780. That means that $49,617 ($59,780 x .83 = $49,617) is available free, and the rest, $10,162 ($59,780 x .17 –pie graph shows 17% in loan is available = $10,162), is available to you in the form of a loan.

So, the total out-of-pocket expense for this school is the initial unmet amount of $0.00 plus the loan amount of $10,162, which equals a total amount of $10,162 – *if* you meet the FAFSA zero EFC and other guidelines and *if* you are awarded all of the available scholarships at the maximum amount.

As I stated in the first college example, keep in mind that this example is just to give you a well-guesstimated ballpark idea of college costs and financial aid distribution. I know, I know, in my example, I figured the total expenses based on the reported on-campus-living expenses, but remember, this is just a demonstration so that you can learn how to run your own numbers. If you had no clue as to how these financial aid awards letters were calculated, now you do!

Again, as I stated in the first college example, keep in mind that, when you call the college to inquire about scholarships, they will tell you, more often than not, that scholarships are need and/or merit based. "Need" is determined by your taxes as discussed above, and FAFSA will determine that for you. "Merit" is driven by your GPA.

Run the numbers

So the technique here is to remember that if you are going on for further education, *do not merely consider the closest college to your home*, especially if you are the type of learner who can utilize an online degree completion program! Furthermore, do not merely look at the college that you think costs less until you run the numbers!

Now it's time to compare the numbers. Remember the formula: **COA-EFC= (NEED/HGP) + (SD) =TC**. I can only utilize portions of this formula since the SD (i.e., student desirability) is unknown. However, look at this eye-popping example:

From these examples alone, we can see that the first college looks like it costs $26,628 a year and the second college looks like it costs $59,780 a year. Up front, I bet that most of you would have chosen the first college. That decision would have cost you $20,570 per year; whereas the second college would have cost you $10,162 per year – less than half the price of the first college! When deciding between schools, make sure you *run the numbers* because now you know how to!

Free money

FYI, make sure that you turn in your FAFSA 1/2/20XX ASAP. Remember: When competing for FAFSA dollars, the early bird gets the worm! Since your new taxes are not yet finished in the beginning of January (when you should be turning in your FAFSA), turn in your FAFSA based on estimated taxes from the year before. Yes, the government allows you to do this! This technique will place you in line for the FAFSA *free* money. Then, when you update your taxes, simply turn in the updated numbers. But this way, you will not lose your place in line for the free money!!!

Poker face

Did you also know that you should apply to seven to 10 colleges? Not only do you avoid putting all your eggs in one basket with this technique, but it provides you with a poker face, so that you seem in demand in the eyes of the college of your choice. Also, when you complete the FAFSA, put the college of your choice in the middle of your list, so you have a poker face here, too. Don't show them all your cards, meaning, don't let them know which college you want to go to.

Why should you do this? If you don't and you make the fatal mistake of only listing *one* college on your FAFSA, the college of your choice will not award you all the FAFSA money to get you to go to there. The college knows – because you told it – that it is the only college that you are looking at spending thousands of dollars at. From the college's perspective, you don't need to be enticed as much to go there, since you already showed them that you have no other college options!

Well gee, if the people that run the college run it like a business – and they do – why should they give you the full amount of free FAFSA money when there is no need for them to compete over your business? Think about it! College, like nursing, is a *business*. That's why you must play poker, don a poker face and make colleges compete for *you*.

Narrow your list

Now that you know how to get the most free money from available sources, I want to remind you to pick colleges that are equal in nature (i.e., they all offer online RN-BSN completion programs; they are all of equal size; they are all in a similar area; etc.). Now, pick the one that gives *you* the most free money!!!

EFC too high?

This is all fine and dandy, but what if you now know that *your EFC* is too high and you do not qualify for FAFSA money? Don't despair! If you do not already have a low EFC you should visit websites such as: WhitePicketCollege.com for more information. Go to the far right tab labeled "Tax and Finance Help." Then go to the tab labeled "Schedule C."

From there, my *highest* recommendation would be to review the information from Sandy Botkin, CPA, Esq. Mr. Botkin is one of 15 CPA/attorneys who has trained IRS agents, so he is someone that you want to learn tax-strategy techniques from! Mr. Botkin's tax-saving techniques and strategies have provided me with sound, realistic and doable tax-savings strategies, which have literally saved me thousands and thousands of dollars over the years. I personally and highly recommend his company. For more information, visit TaxReductionInstitute.com . Utilize coupon code "SAVING" to have 10 percent deducted from the total cost of anything that you purchase.

Avoid student debt

Why do I take the time to talk about how much college costs and how to decrease your cost? Because student loan debt will haunt you forever. If you have any student loan debt, you should pay it off ASAP. But the first step to avoiding large student loan debt later is to avoid incurring a lot of student loan debt now!

Debt is debt, whether the debt is from a credit card or student loan. The difference is that student loan debt can be deducted from your paychecks, your social security checks, etc. if you do not pay it off. Additionally, if you default on your student loans, your RN license can be put in jeopardy, meaning that the license that you worked so hard to obtain – and perhaps even went into debt for – could be pulled and you could be left unable to work. All the while, the student loan debt will continue to haunt you, interest can continue to grow if the loan is in the deferment period, and the problem will become more vicious.

Co-signer caution

If you have had someone co-sign for your private student loan or if you have co-signed for a private student loan, you should put a term life insurance policy for the amount of the loan on the student whose name is on the loan. Make the beneficiary of the term life insurance policy the co-signer of the student loan so that the co-signer, is not stuck with the student loan debt in the event of the student's death.

Student loan debt dies with the death of the student *unless* there is a co-signer. In that case, the debt is shifted to the co-signer, and the debt will not die with the death of the student. YIKES!

This is because private student loans are given by banks, and banks make their own policies. Not all banks forgive the loan debt upon the death of a student when there is a co-signer, even though the co-signer did not benefit from the loan for college. This ultimately means that the loan will not be forgiven. For more information on this subject, please visit

StudentLoanFactsPage.com/418/do-loans-die-when-you-die/#axzz1s1eWzQgD.

Think now

Phew, there is a lot of information in this chapter! I don't mean to overwhelm you, but it is better that you start thinking of some of these issues now, especially if you are still in the process of pursuing a BSN degree. Addressing issues—such as how to create your own internship opportunities, how to make yourself more appealing to potential employers or colleges and how to get the most money from available sources to pay for college—now will help lessen the stress that some nursing graduates face.

Before we move on to the best techniques for applying to a coveted college or nursing position in chapter 4, I would like to address the issue of malpractice protection in chapter 3. This way, you are covered in your internship and other nursing endeavors, as you make your way to your dream nursing job!

Chapter 3:

Safe Nursing

We all have the same amount of time in a day, 24 hours. We all need to somehow earn income to pay for our daily needs, shelter, food, clothing, etc. We all need to sleep. Of our 24 hours, most people work eight hours a day, not to mention the time people take for breaks, plus the time it takes to commute to and from work. In addition, most people desire eight hours of sleep within that same timeframe.

If you spend a third of your 24-hour day working and as much as a third of your precious day sleeping, why then would you not protect what you work so hard for in the first place, your livelihood and income? If you protect yourself and your income, you will not waste the remaining eight hours or third of your day by fighting to protect what you have worked so hard for.

Think about it. When you choose the nursing profession, you are at a higher risk of assuming "problems" in the workplace than most because you are, after all, dealing with people and medicine! Nursing school is not easy, so why are you not protecting what you worked so hard to get, namely your license?

Protect yourself as an intern

Remember, if you are volunteering as an intern, using the technique that I showed you for setting up your own internship, you are not doing this as a student of your school / college / university. Therefore, you do not have any malpractice coverage. But this is no big deal. If you hop on Google and look up nursing malpractice insurance sites you will find that you can pick up malpractice coverage for an RN student nurse rather inexpensively. The cost will vary state to state. So, how much does it run? Well, as an example, on one site I found, as of July 2012 in Illinois, it costs less than $40.00 per year to get quite a bit of malpractice coverage. Look up your particular state, determine how much malpractice insurance you need and decide if the internships you create are worth pursuing from a financial perspective.

Protect yourself as a nurse

If you already are a RN, I would still highly suggest that you have your own malpractice insurance, separate from what is offered through your place of employment. As our healthcare system is changing, nurses are becoming a growing target of malpractice charges. For instance, the third edition of a text entitled Ethics and Issues in Contemporary Nursing by Margaret A. Burkhardt and Alvita K. Nathaniel states that "traditional errors such as burns, falls, and medication errors seem to be more common than in the past.

This leads to the speculation that negligent actions are a direct result of increased stress in the workplace and decreased morale, which together lead to the overall effect of distracting nurses from focusing clearly on individual patients" (page 169). Insightful.

If your employer informs you that you are covered under their malpractice insurance policy and that you do not need your own malpractice insurance, I would ask, "Why then do physicians who are employed by the same hospital have their own malpractice insurance?" Things that make you go hmm.

There are old-school thinkers in nursing who will tell you that you do not need your own malpractice insurance. Those people who have an older mindset will tell you that your employer will cover you. I would encourage you to talk to an attorney and ask for his or her opinion. From what I know, I would rather spend a tiny bit on insurance to protect the earnings that I have worked so hard for than to be caught off guard without enough coverage under an employer's policy for whatever reason.

Nurses and malpractice suits

The truth is that in 2012 and beyond, nurses are being named in lawsuits, and individual nurses are being held responsible rather than the hospital or facility that employs them. If you rely upon your employer, then you are 100 percent at his or her mercy. For instance, your employer may say that you are covered but there are certain caveats. Let's say that you did one thing that did not comply with the employer's policies and procedures. This may lead to a call from your employer's attorney, saying that you are now not covered under the employer's medical malpractice insurance.

The old school thinkers will say that in a lawsuit, people go after deep pockets and that is why you do not need to personally have coverage. Really? Perhaps these old-school thinkers have not looked at the news, listened to the news or talked to people about anything other than the weather lately because first of all, we live in the most litigious society there is. You have more than a 30-percent chance of being sued!

If those old-school thinkers are touting that the deep pockets that people go after are those with millions and millions of dollars, ask them to explain why people sue others for $10,000 or less all day long in the Illinois small claims court system, not to mention the small claims court financial cut-off amount for other states! If people do not sue for small amounts, then why are there so many small claims court TV shows such as Judge Judy, People's Court, Judge Greg Mathis Show, Judge Joe Brown Show, Judge Hatchett, etc.?

Maybe these old-school thinkers who believe that lawsuits are only brought against those with deep pockets need a wake-up call! This is a false belief! That's why I point out all the small-claims-court shows that are on TV. Your pockets may not be very deep yet, but you are still at risk of being named a defendant in a lawsuit.

Employers

I ask you this: How has that old way of thinking worked out for those that rely on their employer to keep them employed until they can retire? There are reports everywhere in the news of people being laid off just a few years before they are set to retire from a company for which they worked as loyal employees for more than 30 years. Now let me ask you this: If you have seen this type of thing happen around you, then why put yourself at risk by thinking that your employer will be loyal to you when push comes to shove? What makes you so special? You are not. You are a number. Sad, but true. So now that you know better, do better. I greatly encourage you to protect yourself.

> **"You must constantly ask yourself these questions: Who am I around? What are they doing to me? What have they got me reading? What have they got me saying? Where do they have me going? What do they have me thinking? And most important, what do they have me becoming? Then ask yourself the big question: Is that okay?"**
>
> -- Jim Rohn

Protect your identity

The biggest area of coverage that I suggest that you get if you are a student, if you are an RN, or, heck, even if you are not in nursing at all is identity theft monitoring with full restoration coverage and legal services.

Why? Think about it. When you go to the hospital as a nursing student, quite often the patients/clients do not even realize that you are a student. Sadly. They next assume that since you are "working" at a healthcare facility that you have a paid position, as well as insurance. And in order to get a paid position, they assume that you have the proper legal documents to work in the United

States, as well as coveted medical insurance. Now, this may or may not be true, but it is likely that your entire name is printed on your ID badge ripe for the taking.

You know, it does not take much for people to take your name, look you up online and use the information that is in cyber world to steal your social security number, medical identity and other forms of identity theft. How do you even know if this is happening or not if you do not have a monitoring service in place?

Worse yet, if you only have your credit report monitored, how do you restore your identity when a breech occurs? All forms of identity theft – medical, social security, driver's license, financial, criminal and character – have been listed for the 12th straight year by the Federal Trade Commission, FTC, as a major concern for Americans, according to an article in money.msn.com. There are more complaints about identity theft than any other type of fraud or scam.

Oh let me guess….you think a credit lock or a credit freeze is what I'm speaking of? No, those make your life miserable for when you do want further credit extended. Do you fully understand what a credit lock or a credit freeze actually does? A credit lock or a credit freeze simply means that the credit bureaus cannot inform someone of your current credit score to then extend credit lending from. A lock for a freeze simply stops the ability to obtain new credit based on your current score! A credit lock or credit freeze does not stop the ability for you, or someone else, to use your name for multiple other purposes. You see, if you have a credit lock or a credit freeze in place, then lending off of your current credit score is not allowed, but there are places that do not pull your current score and do lend! Examples? How about renting a home from a small private investor or mom & pop place, obtaining new utility service, obtaining phone service in your name, gaining employment (unless a credit check is required to obtain a job), etc. A credit lock or freeze will not stop existing accounts, such as credit cards, to be utilized. See what I mean! A credit lock or credit freeze simply helps to stop the opening of new accounts that require a credit check – nothing more. Do not fall for the false sense of security with a credit lock or a credit freeze as that is not a true mean of protection.

Let me ask you, are you working hard to become an RN or did you work hard to become an RN? Then protect that license! When someone steals your identity, they can hurt your nursing license. Once your license is compromised, your income is compromised. Do not wait.

Not having an identity-theft monitoring and restoration service is as crazy as hopping onto your bank account via the internet while using a public computer that does not have any virus protection. D-U-M-B.

Personally, I exclusively endorse identity theft services that offer additional legal services too, since you can utilize the legal help with daily life questions about anything such as traffic tickets, mortgage questions, divorce decrees, student loans, immigration issues, wills, etc. Visit NursingCareerProfessionals.com or contact me directly at Info@NursingCareerProfessionals.com to learn more about this service so that you can be protected (United States and Canada residents only. Citizenship not required; residency of either country is required).

Pot of gold

Think of having access to legal services from another perspective, as well. Once you have malpractice insurance – either insurance that you pay for yourself and/or insurance that the hospital / employer pays for – you have a so-called pot of gold that you need to protect. Who is able to protect your pot of gold? Not you! You are not an attorney; you are a nurse! Keep in mind that when you are named in a lawsuit, the malpractice insurance is only good once the award from the lawsuit is awarded. Well, what happens before that? Who will you talk to if you have any legal questions?

Let me remind you that you will get sued. People are sue happy and are frequently looking for money. Nowadays, nurses are being named in lawsuits left and right. Heck, worse yet, what do you do if the lawsuit awards more than the pot of gold that you have? Too late then. To avoid all of this, just get legal coverage now. By the way, identity theft and legal coverage for you and your entire family costs less than $1.00 a day – total for everyone in the family, not just for one person! I know, this is a big ah-ha moment and a no-brainer.

Are you wondering what kind of attorney you will have access to for $1.00 a day? Let me simply put it this way, what type of physician do you have access to for a $20.00 co-pay? Exactly! This concept is the same for the legal world as health insurance is for the medical world. Again, simply something you should not be without. You need to protect your license, yourself and your family.

Additionally, you can also utilize the service to create a living will, as well as a durable power of attorney for healthcare. These are the same documents that you learn about in school and that you ask your patients/clients about all the time. These are the same documents that all the financial gurus tell you to have in place! Shockingly, eight out of 10 people do not have these documents in place! But now that the main cost issue and the need have been addressed, it is part of my revolutionary nursing mission to change this sad fact.

Financial advisors such as Suze Orman, Dave Ramsey and other big financial gurus constantly mention the need for people to have these documents in place, and I am blazing a trail in the nursing world to show you how to get these done in order to protect you and your family!

For further information, please visit www.NursingCareerProfessionals.com or email me at info@NursingCareerProfessionals.com. You will find access to different types of top-rated attorneys that you may need for possible questions about a will, speeding tickets, student loans, children or dependents, debt collection issues, a house note or landlord/tenant agreement, employment, immigration questions, etc.

Now that you know how to protect yourself, while in school, as an RN and beyond, let's move on to chapter 4. In chapter 4, I will show you how to get noticed when applying for a competitive and coveted nursing position.

Chapter 4:

Make Your Application Stand Out

Through my daughter's violin playing, I was introduced to Mark Wood, a violinist who truly stands out as a violin player.

Mark Wood is one of the best examples that I can share to illustrate how important it is to set yourself apart from the competition, while staying true to your profession. Mark Wood is in the music world, but by taking a look at Mark's life, you will quickly learn how you can spotlight yourself within the nursing profession.

Mark Wood is a world-renowned electric violinist, an Emmy-winning composer and an international recording artist, and he is widely acknowledged as the premier electric-rock violinist of his generation. Of course he did not start out that way.

Mark studied at Tanglewood and attended the Juilliard School of Music on a full scholarship, which he left to pursue his vision of bringing rock violin into the mainstream. His first release was widely hailed as the quintessential rock violin record.

For 13 years, he was the string master of the Trans-Siberian Orchestra, receiving two platinum and three gold records for his work with them. He has also toured and performed with Billy Joel, Celine Dion, Dee Snider's Van Helsing's Curse, Lenny Kravitz, Steve Vai, Roger Daltry of the Who and Jewel. Mark has been a featured guest on *The Tonight Show* with Jay Leno and has had articles written about him in the *New York Times*, *USA Today* and *Time Magazine*, among others.

Mark plays symphonic rock, hard rock and heavy metal on a violin. He plays an electric violin that was made from Wood Violins, a company the he founded that makes revolutionary, custom-built, unique electric violins.

When you think of a violin, what type of music do you associate with it? Most people would say classical music … unless they have met Mark.

When you think of a nurse, what picture comes to mind? Most people would think of someone in scrubs, in a hospital setting … unless they have met me.

Mark has become a friend to our family, and he is one of many who have inspired us throughout the years. In fact, due to his inspirations, we have two of these violins in our household. And although I do not play either, my husband and daughter do!

Be a rock star

How can you take this information and use it to help you stand out as a nurse? Mark Wood has taken a classical instrument, the violin, and made it appeal to a wider array of people by expanding the type of music which is played on such an instrument. Mark's inspirations have led me to think differently about what I do. As a nurse, it is important to appeal to a wider array of employers and health care providers than in the past.

You too have the potential to stand out, and I now encourage you to do the same in your career. Your nursing employment application is the first step. So, let me share specific techniques with you that will allow you make the most of your potential to become a rock star in the nursing world!

In this chapter, I show you how to get noticed among a sea of applicants, all applying to the same coveted nursing position. I give you some tips to keep in mind while filling out job applications, as well as some pointers to follow after you have completed your application for an available nursing position.

Keep some things private

These days when you apply for a position it is usually online. Since this is a quick and easy way to apply for your dream nursing job, you may be tempted to instantly start filling out job applications left and right. OK, stop. There are a few things that you need to know before you fill out a job application, whether it is online or in person.

First, contact your employment attorney and find out what type of questions an employer in your state is legally allowed to ask on a job application. *Many* of you give out way too much information – information that the employer is thrilled to receive if you are offering it, since he or she is not legally allowed to ask you for it!

Refer to chapter 3 for information about how to gain access to an attorney for a relatively inexpensive cost, and additionally, you can go to NursingCareerProfessionals.com for further insight.

Information better left unsaid

What are examples of information that you should not offer a prospective employer? Hmm, how about the obvious old-school ones? Clearly, no one can ask you if you are pregnant, but if you volunteer that information, that is a different story. Clearly no one can ask you if you are married, but if you volunteer that information, that is a different story.

Another example of something that an employer is not allowed to ask you on a job application, in an interview, etc. is your age. So if there is a field on your online job application, or even on a hard copy, that asks what year you finished college, you should *not* fill that out!

In fact, you should not list the year that you completed college on your resume, or on your Facebook page! The same thing goes for the year you completed high school. Oh, and nix your full birth date from showing up on Facebook too. Just list the day and month of your birth. WHY? To avoid age discrimination!

No assumptions

This technique helps level the playing field. Think about it. If you are young, someone could assume that you are not as stable of a job candidate as an older person, that you will be partying more, that you are going to get married and have a child, or whatever. Again, this is an *assumption,* but *you* gave the employer the chance to let his or her brain run wild with false ideas because you told the person your graduation dates. Now that person is trying to figure out how old you are.

Also, the employer may make some ridiculous assumptions by knowing your graduation dates. For instance, you could be 42, having just graduated from community college, after having attended any sort of college for the first time at age 40. But more than likely, the person that reads your resume and job application will assume that you went to college at age 18 and are now 20 years old.

If you do point out to the employer that you are older, you also run the risk that the employer will assume that you have too many other obligations to make you a qualified job candidate, that you will not learn quickly, that you can only work certain days and will not work weekends, etc, etc, etc. Again, these are false ideas, but there is *no* need to give a prospective employer a chance to let his or her brain run wild with false assumptions that you have no control over. So, nix those dates! The important point is that you either have a degree or will have a degree soon!!

Leave off your application

Other information that you should not supply on a job application is the amount of income that you made at your previous job. Why would you tell a prospective employer that? You expect to receive nothing less than a fair-market, competitive offer, right? Well then, it does not matter what you made at your prior position, even if that position was in the same field.

If you are completing an online application that does not allow you to leave the "previous income" field blank, you can put in a number that is so odd that the employer will think it is a typo or fictitious amount. Now some of you may be thinking, "The employer will not consider my application if I do not fill out every blank field on the job application or if I put in really low numbers." If this is the case with you, I ask: Do you really want to work for that low of pay? If yes, then fill out that information. But if you want to receive a salary that is competitive like you deserve, then leave that information blank.

After applying

Next technique: Now that you have filled out the application online, I recommend that you print out a hard copy of your resume and slide it under the hiring manager's door! Oh yeah, I *did* just say that!

First of all, let me remind you that it is likely that you are seeking a hospital position. Do you realize that a hospital is open 24/7/365? So call the hospital during an off shift and find out who the manager of whatever department you applied to work in is, whether the department is, NICU, OR, ED, Tele, or whatever. If the operator does not know who the manager is, ask to be transferred to that department. Then simply ask the person that answers the phone who the manager is. Next, write down the manager's name.

Now, *go* to the hospital. *Go* to that department. I recommend going during an off shift or weekend. Keep in mind that your goal is not to speak with the hiring manager face to face right now, but to get her or him to see your resume. So, slide your resume under the door of the unit manager's office or ask the staff to do it for you.

Now call and leave a message on the manager's phone line by calling the operator again. Keep in mind that when you leave your message, you should first let the manager know how she or he can benefit from hiring you. After you have done that, *then* leave your name.

People must learn what is in it for them first, *then* they will keep listening. That is why you must say your name *last*. Hearing your name does not offer any insight as to how you can help a potential employer. What you want a potential employer to hear *first* – and what he or she wants to hear *first* – is what you have to offer. For example, you can say:

"I have great news for you, Manager 'X'! I know that I can help you with your budgeting problem on the unit, so I have left a copy of my resume in your office (or I had Nurse 'X' put a copy in your office), as well as an online application with HR. My name is 'XXXXXXX' and I will follow up with you in 'X' amount of days, or you may reach me at the contact information that is listed on my resume."

Remember, if you say that you are going to follow up in 'X' amount of days, be sure you do!

This technique is similar to what I have personally learned from Tony Parinello. Tony is the author of *Selling to VITO, the Very Important Top Officer: Get to the Top. Get to the Point. Get to the Sale*. (Tony has also personally trained more than 2.5 million salespeople, and a majority of business people in the Fortune 500 companies. In other words, his techniques work!) Well in this case, the "sale" that you are trying to make is *you!* I have not only read his book, but I have personally taken his course and realized, yet again, that nursing is a business. Thus, I have utilized his business strategies, but I have put a nursing spin on them for your benefit.

Get noticed

Why do I suggest doing this? The answer is to think about who has the short position on the unit. It is the unit manager. Who will have budget issues when the other staff RNs pick up overtime to fill the shortage? The unit manager. Who has a fire lit under her or him to fill any open positions? The unit manager. Yet you applied to the Human Resources department and are simply *waiting* for a person in that department who is not under much pressure to fill the position to notice you? Really?

What do you have to lose? After all, this technique that I am offering you does show initiative. It shows that you communicate well. It shows that you see the bigger picture since you pointed out the budgeting concerns. Think about it! Dare to be different! Or your other option is to apply to HR and *hope* that they look at your resume.

You are passionate about wanting to land a position as a RN. You have the potential to *be* an amazing nurse, so why not go for it? Remember what Mark Wood has taught me and my family, which is to be different and to stand apart from the rest. What *if* these techniques work for you? People who think and act differently are the ones who rise to the top! Go for it!

> **"Knowing you need to make a change isn't enough. You've got to find the guts to do it."**
>
> -- Robert Kiyosaki

Again, now is the time to ask yourself: Will I be up to the challenge? Will I become successful? Will I be as good as or better than those who came before me? In order to succeed, you must build your *knowledge*, take *action* and overcome your *fear*. You must take the knowledge that I have given you – how to get noticed while applying for a competitive nursing position – and combine that with action to land your dream job!

In this chapter, we have discussed how to stand out when applying for a competitive nursing position. Next, in chapter 5, I would like to discuss a few things to keep in mind when deciding *where* to work as a nurse.

Chapter 5:

The Rise and Fall of Incomes

A family friend of ours landed his first marketing position straight out of college about three years back. He was in his mid 20s at the time. He got a company car, benefits, etc., and he now has a mortgage on a home. Although the vast majority of his circle of friends and family would tout that he has a wonderful position, that he is stable and that life for him is good, I see things differently.

Why? Most people only see a small fraction of the bigger picture. Many people would tell this young man that he is stable, when actually he is in the *riskiest scenario*. The way I see it, this young man only has *one* position to draw experience from.

In my opinion, he should seek another opportunity, which would not only build his experience base, but would probably help his pay skyrocket. In my opinion, by staying in one position, he is playing Russian Roulette.

When his number is called in today's world of downsizing, he has so much to lose: a home, his company car and his only position of experience to draw from. Not to mention that as time continues, he will eventually *have* to have his own medical insurance coverage (although at his current age, he could still remain on his parents' policy). All of this, and I have not yet addressed his limited pay.

So you can avoid suffering this same risky fate, I will show you how to dramatically advance your pay in the first several years of your career when there is an available "income rise" to capitalize on. This way, you can better financially prepare for your future. You see, there is a way for our subject to rise above the challenges, just as there is a way for you to rise above any challenges that you may experience in your nursing career. You simply need to see a bigger picture.

Income roller coaster

In this chapter, I would like to discuss the rise, plateau and decline of RN income, as well as provide a technique to overcome this challenge.

I have been a nursing instructor at the college and university level for many years and have found that, sadly, most nursing students are only being groomed for a stereotypical registered nursing career within the confines of a hospital, long-term care facility or doctor's office. But because this is the case, this is where we will begin: with a look at the income potential in this sector.

There is a rise, plateau and decline of income in this role as a staff RN in these types of facilities that I stated above.

Pay ceilings

It has always been interesting to me that hospitals blatantly advertise their "New Grad RN" base pay rates, yet fail to advertise what they pay people with experience. Think about it. Look through any nursing journal or on any job site, and you will see firsthand what I mean.

Why do hospitals fail to advertise pay rates for experienced nurses? Each hospital is competing against the next local hospital for customers/clients/patients. Therefore, it is in the hospital's best interest to have whomever they qualify/quantify as the best nurses on their nursing staff. And the easiest way for a hospital to win the attention of the best nurses is through financial enticement. Thus, advertising only the entry level rate of pay is a way of leveling the playing field.

Once a new graduate nurse is hired, her or his pay increases over time; however, this pay rate will not keep increasing.

For example, it seems fair to say that a staff RN working 40 hours a week (before considering shift differential, weekend differential or call pay) is not making six figures at her/his job. Would you agree? So what this means is that over time, say 30 or more years, the pay rate is leveling off for a staff RN. There is a pay ceiling.

Decreasing pay

What is even scarier is that a staff RN's pay rate can also decrease over time. In today's economic downturn, people agree to take a cut in pay verses losing her or his job. The pay cut can be reflected as a decrease in one's pay rate per hour or even as a cut in the hours per week that an RN is scheduled to work.

When a hospital faces financial losses that occur when patients or potential customers do not have health insurance due to job losses of their own, or that occur due to cutbacks on the government Medicare or Medicaid systems, then the hospital looks to make cutbacks. Keep in mind that one of the biggest overhead expenses, if not *the* biggest overhead expense, is staffing. Thus, cutbacks to staffing positions or scheduled hours can serve to decrease the overall rate of pay for a staff RN.

The following excerpt from an article entitled the "Top 5 Challenges Facing Nursing in 2012" by Rebecca Hendren, published in *HealthLeaders Media* in November 2011, highlights these issues: "Nursing knows that hiring freezes and layoffs are a constant threat and healthcare organizations are forced to put cost cutting at the top of the agenda in 2012. As the largest budget in the organization, nursing is an easy target."

Your second position

Given all these factors leading to the plateau and possible decline of staff RN pay rates over time, how do you capitalize on the initial increase of income that the staff RN position offers new hires? Let me show you!

Pretend that you live in an area where every hospital is equal in esteem. We will say they are all Level II facilities for this hypothetical scenario. Suppose that every unit, specialty unit and medical surgical unit wants to hire *you*, the new grad. Also, suppose that the hospitals do not care what your education background as an RN is, meaning that they do not give more weight to a master's or bachelor's degree than to an associate's degree. *Everything* is considered equally. Now suppose that the pay is $20.00 per hour at every hospital and that the shift differentials and weekend differentials are the same. The only difference between these scenarios is the distance to your home.

Next, imagine that you apply to all the hospitals and that every hospital offers you the same position, which calls for three 12-hour days, constituting a full-time position. Don't forget that all the hospitals are offering the same pay rate, $20.00 an hour. [By taking the hourly pay, $20.00, multiplying that by the total number of full-time working hours in a year (i.e., 40 hours a week x 52 weeks in a year = 2080 total hours in a year), you will arrive at the total pay per year.] So, $20.00 x 2080 total hours = $41,600 in income per year.

Location choice

Which hospital would you pick and why? Think this out before you answer too quick!

X Hospital ABC	**X Hospital DEF**
X YOU LIVE HERE	
	X Hospital GHI
X Hospital JKL	
X Hospital MNO	
	X Hospital PQR
X Hospital STU	
X Hospital XYZ	

Carmen Kosicek, RN, MSN

I am guessing that you picked a hospital close to your home. That is exactly what most people pick in this scenario. I understand this rationale given today's expensive gas prices and the resulting need to cut down on a driving commute.

So let's say that you choose hospital ABC because it is the closest one to your home. And let's say that after one year goes by, your boss is doing your review and raves, raves, raves about your performance. They *love* you at hospital ABC!

Pay raise expectations

How much of a raise are you expecting since, clearly, you are a rock-star nurse? Keep in mind that you are making a little more than $40,000 per year in this scenario.

Do you think that your raise will be $4,000 or 10 percent? Definitely not. How about half of that, $2,000 or 5 percent? More than likely, another *no*.

Most raises are in the range of 2.5 percent. So if you take an annual pay of $40,000 and multiply that by 0.025, which equals $1,000, and divide that by your hourly rate of $20.00, you will get an eye-popping 50-cent raise per hour. Yup. That is it. You will get a pay raise of about $1,000 after working one year as the unit's rock-star nurse. Aside from the disappointing amount of the pay raise in this scenario, it is more important to focus on that last sentence. And what is so magical about that last sentence?? Go ahead and look at it. ...It says that you have *worked for one year*. What that really means is that you have *experience*!

www.NursingCareerProfessionals.com | 66

After seeing the raise that hospital ABC is offering you after one year of impressive service, perhaps you now decide that the short commute time and amount of gas that you are saving isn't worth it for the $0.50 raise per hour that you received. You decide that you need and are worth more money, so you apply farther away from home at hospital XYZ.

Parlay your experience

The hospitals continue to advertise to new RN grads with a beginning pay of $20.00 an hour. But now that you have experience and make $20.50 an hour, what do you think hospital XYZ will offer you? Remember, you won't need as long of an orientation timeframe because you have some experience under your belt, and that is a *huge* savings for the hospital. I would easily bet that you will be offered something in the range of $23.00 to $24.00 an hour.

Nice! This means that you just jumped the pay scale by $5,200.00 to $7,280.00 a year with an hourly raise of $2.50 to $3.50 an hour. (A raise of $2.50 per hour x 2080 total working hours in one year = a raise of $5,200 per year. A raise of $3.50 per hour x 2080 total working hours in one year = a raise of $7,280.00 per year). Wow! That could pay for a lot!

Or think about it this way: moving from hospital ABC to hospital XYZ means that you can choose to work fewer hours and make the same amount of money, since your initial pay rate is higher at hospital XYZ. For example, you can work from 253 to 355 hours *less* at the new hospital, depending on how much higher your rate of pay is at hospital XYZ (using the range of pay that we've established for our scenario).

More importantly, think about how many years of *time* it would have taken for you to increase your base pay if you had chosen to stay at hospital ABC.

Go for it! Challenge yourself in your nursing career. Being up for a challenge or perhaps a move from a comfortable situation will help make you more successful in your nursing career! Now that you know what to do, it is time for you to take action!

> **"He who is not courageous enough to take risks will accomplish nothing in life."**
>
> -- Muhammad Ali

The farther job

Surprisingly, choosing hospital ABC because it is closest to your home may not be the best choice, from both a financial and professional perspective. I am frequently asked why I recommend that someone choose a position that is farthest away from the person's home. It's simple. Being farther away will entice you to leave after you have gained experience.

You see, we all get comfortable at a job when we know the people around us, know how to do things and are in a routine. Financially speaking, being comfortable may have been alright for our parents' generation and before, but it is not working that way anymore.

In today's economic environment, the problem with getting too comfortable is that if you choose to stay at the same job for 30 or more years and do not learn different ways to do things, what will you do if or when there are job layoffs? Be mindful, this is an unfortunate reality that many face today. When you are downsized, where will you go? Who will want to hire you if you only know one way of doing something? The saying is, "You cannot teach an old dog new tricks," right?

Times have changed since our parents were in the workforce; it is likely that your position will be downsized at one time or another, so prepare for it. In today's times, it is best to build a broad base of experience, so I highly recommend that you build this base *now* when you don't need it. That way, you have it to fall back on later when you do need it.

Let's capitalize on what you can do *now* to make your base of knowledge strong and more diverse for the future. Let's make the sort of money in nursing that the business world has been making for quite some time! Ladies and gentlemen, blending nursing with a strong business sense is just the beginning.

How long to stay

How long should you stay? One to two years is key for your first staff nursing position. Also, it is imperative to keep in mind that it really isn't about the first position, meaning don't get wrapped up in how much the hospital pays. Instead, it is about the experience. Clearly, you see that by moving to the next hospital, your pay will most likely increase. The experience is the most important part of your first 1 to 2 years at this first position.

One of my recent clinical students, "Judith," began her job hunt after we had reviewed this technique of parlaying one's first nursing experience into a new position and higher pay. She quickly learned that she was living in a flooded area – an area experiencing more nurse applicants than nursing positions – the north side of Chicago, Illinois. Judith had not seen any nurse openings in her area, but she had seen a position offered out of state. However, Judith told me that after realizing that the pay was low, she would not consider the out-of-state position – even though the facility was welcoming new graduates.

I pointed out to her that the cost of living was much less in the other state and that this needed to be factored into her analysis. But of greater importance was the fact that if she took a position outside her flooded area, she could get in the door and start working an average of 6 to 9 months sooner than if she were to stay in the flooded area and wait for a position to open. Furthermore, once she could gain needed nursing experience, she could hop back to the flooded state, whose hospitals would then willingly accept her because of her recent experience. And now, her pay would skyrocket! In this scenario, her pay might even surpass what it would have been if she had chosen to stay and wait for a job.

It really does not matter if the difference in nursing positions is $10.00 an hour because *you will not be staying* at that job; that is my point. Your first nursing job is about the experience. Don't get wrapped up in the numbers. Instead, look for the job that will provide you with the experience that you need for the next position that you really want!

All this became clear to Judith. She decided that once she graduates, she is going to position herself to move to an area that isn't flooded, grab a hold of a specialty position, work it for one to two years, and allow that experience to skyrocket her career!

Moving is smart

So, let's talk about moving. I know, I know, you don't think you can go. Well, let's see if you can afford *not* to go. And if you really cannot go, encourage those who can to move so it will increase your odds of landing a coveted position, since there will be fewer candidates for those local positions!

Let's pretend that a set of twins, Stephania and Eliza, have recently graduated from nursing school and have entered into a job market that is experiencing a nursing flood. They both have the exact same background of work experience as student nurses, and they both have student loan debt of $25,000 each. Let's pretend that they both graduated in the December graduating class.

By the time their nursing school reports to the state in which they live and have graduated from that they are able to sit for the RN State Boards, two months have passed. Finally, they receive notice that they are able to schedule and sit for their RN State Board exam.

Stephania and Eliza pass the Boards on the first try. It then takes one to two weeks for the results to arrive at their home.

Have you been adding up the weeks here? More likely than not, their graduation date was before Christmas. It was probably the third week of December. Why am I pointing this out? Most likely, their student loan repayment plans kick in six months from the date that they *graduated.* They could have loans that require interest payments now or at the six-month-post-graduation mark. Do you clearly see that even if everything goes smoothly, they are already two-and-a-half to three months past graduation when they can even *apply* for a nursing position? Remember, this is if everything goes smoothly!

So, Stephania decides to apply for positions in Illinois in the flooded Chicagoland nursing job market. Eliza decides to apply for positions in Florida. They used Indeed.com to find available positions.

Two weeks go by, Stephania has not heard anything from any hospital, and neither has Eliza. They step up the number of applications that they send to numerous facilities, let's say 20 each.

Two more weeks pass, Stephania still has not heard anything, but Eliza has two interviews. Eliza then lands a position and moves south. In our timeline, it is late April. It possibly could be even later, but the point is that it has been at least four months since graduation. And in two months, the dreaded student loan payments start.

Eliza starts working. Stephania is still job hunting. In a flooded market, the average time that it takes a nurse to obtain her or his first position is six to nine months or more *after* passing RN Boards. This means that in a flooded market, it will take the average nurse eight to 11 months or more to obtain a job after graduation. Sure, a few will land positions before that time, but most do not.

True, if she does not have an income yet, Stephania can put the student loan on deferment, but, really, that is simply postponing the inevitable and the interest is likely accruing. When a loan is deferred, the payments are postponed. Some scenarios allow the interest to be deferred as well, but what if it isn't? That is right, the overall debt continues to grow!

If it takes Stephania six to nine months or more to land a job while Eliza is already working, do you see how Eliza will be nearing her one-year-of-experience mark in a few more months, ready to increase her income dramatically? Yet by this same point, Stephania will – if she is lucky – only have a obtained a few months of experience in this game. Remember, it is likely that Stephania will *not* have specialty unit experience, but Eliza will. This is a *huge* difference.

At the end of the 12-month mark, Eliza decides to move *back* to Chicagoland. This time when she applies to hospitals, she has *experience. Huge* difference. If she highlights her experience well, she will have interviews booked with organizations in the flooded area within a few weeks of applying.

Back to the income scenario, Eliza will now be able to increase her pay dramatically in comparison to what her hourly pay would have been if she had stayed at her current position. She can easily jump the pay scale by a few years! Additionally, on Eliza's resume, her move will make sense and not make her appear as a "job hopper." This is because she is moving from one state to another, versus going to another hospital in the same market. Strategically speaking, this is a genius move for her career.

Avoiding a nursing flood

Do these ideas really work? Here is a true story.

"April" was a Bachelor-Degree-seeking-student nurse of mine in 2010. She lived in downtown Chicago and only wanted a position in OB. After graduation as her loan payment was kicking in, she frantically phoned me for help. She had been applying and applying and applying for nursing positions, but no one would give her a chance to get "experience." In addition, this was in a *hugely* competitive market, downtown Chicago! Sadly, as I pointed out to her, it was and still is a hugely competitive market with a nursing flood.

Again, April insisted on a position in OB. After my lead, April applied out of state. She chose Texas. Straight out of school, she landed a full-time position on a specialty unit. April moved. She ended up being cross-trained at a Level II facility, and after a year, she additionally picked up a registry position at a Level I facility. Brilliant move! You see, she is broadening her base!

Just before the two-year mark, April decided she wanted to return to Chicago where her family was. After highlighting her experience appropriately on her resume, April, who was from out of state, landed more than three interviews at various hospitals downtown Chicago in the same week! To say the least, she was thrilled!

Fast-forward to one week after the interviews:. April texted me to inform me that she was offered *two* full-time positions, both in downtown Chicago – one at Northwestern and one at Rush!

She asked what she should do. I told her to take *both* positions! She had already accepted the Northwestern full-time position one day after she interviewed, so I recommended that she pick up PRN at Rush! It is always better to build a bigger base, after all!

Was April up to the challenge? *Yes!* Will she become successful? *Yes!* Was April choosing to be as good as or better than those who came before her? *Yes!* And you can be, too.

In order to succeed, you must build your *knowledge*, take *action* and overcome your *fear*. You must take the knowledge that I have given you – how to overcome RN income and employment trends – and combine that with action to land your dream job!

In this chapter, we discussed the rise, plateau, and decline of RN income, as well as how to think outside the box in regard to the challenge of landing a nursing position in a flooded market – especially as the student-loan time bomb is ticking. I have offered you information regarding how the nursing pay system works, as well as illustrated techniques for gaining experience and using your current amount of income to drive a greater amount of income at your next place of employment.

In the following chapter, I will explain why certain areas of the country are regarded as "flooded" with potential nurses who are vying for limited positions. I will discuss how to analyze a market so you will be able to tell if there is a flood, and I will give you specific techniques for landing a nursing position in a flooded area. Additionally, alternative nursing options to typical hospital offerings will be discussed.

Chapter 6:

Your First Job

Job growth for RNs is increasing at a staggering rate. According to the U.S. Department of Labor at bls.gov, RN job growth is set to increase by 26 percent from 2010 to 2020. This is considered a faster-than-average increase of growth in comparison to all other occupations!

You have probably heard this good news, this positive statistic about RNs. So then, why is it that you still feel anxious or skeptical about landing your first nursing position? Why are you concerned that this may be a challenge? Why are those around you not landing RN positions right and left?

The answer is that you are probably trying to find nursing work in a flooded market. *Grand.* But is there hope? Yes! Not only is there hope that you will be able to land a nursing position in a flooded market, but you have finally connected with someone who can guide you step by step and show you how exactly to land your first RN position, no matter where you are located.

Flooded areas

There are several things to think about when trying to land a coveted nursing position. As we have already discussed, *where* to work is a significant factor in easily being able to land a nursing position. Of course, as I have previously mentioned, it is ideal if you can move out of a flooded area for a relatively short period of time, gain experience in a readily available nursing position in a non-flooded area, and eventually use that experience and rate of income to land a coveted (and well-paid) position in whatever area you wish. However, I realize that this strategy may not be an option for everyone. So I would like to discuss why certain areas are flooded and how to overcome this obstacle if you must work in a flooded area.

How flooding happens

Let's take the flooded area that I lived and worked in as an example. For just shy of 35 years, I lived in the Chicagoland southwest suburbs. Chicagoland, as it's known by locals, is made up of the metropolitan areas of Chicago proper and its surrounding sprawling suburbs. So, Chicagoland sounds like it must have a competitive job market, right? Right. In reports by Infoplease.com, Chicago was ranked third in a list of the top 50 most populous cities in the United States in 2010, with an estimated population of more than 2.6 million. Chicago came in right behind New York and Los Angeles, which were the top two most populous cities in the U.S., respectively.

Thus, nursing growth is on the rise, *but* there is also a "flood" of RNs in Chicagoland. There are nursing programs everywhere, and they are quickly cranking out nurses left and right. Often, the wait to be admitted into the nursing programs in the area is several years long – *if* the school even admits that there is a waiting period. Sometimes, a school will require you to reapply to a nursing program on a semester-by-semester basis to avoid acknowledging that there is a bona fide wait list. Remember that nursing is a business, and the business side knows the importance of how something is presented!

In the far southwestern suburbs of Chicago, there are more than eight RN programs within a 30-minute radius of the main city, and each program graduates RNs twice a year with an average of 60 RNs per graduating class! I hope that this insight gives you a grasp of the potential volume of new nurses that are in a flooded market.

Economic environment

It would be ideal if the nurses who are already working in these flooded markets were retiring, but they are not. They are continuing to work because of the poor economic environment.

Perhaps a nurse of retirement age has a spouse who was downsized a few years before his or her retirement, and the nursing spouse must now provide the household's main source of income or healthcare benefits for both partners. Or perhaps a married couple is padding their retirement accounts to make up for any financial shortcomings they may have suffered when the market fell a few years ago. Perhaps a married couple is not able to sell their house at a profit anymore, yet that is where they were thinking their retirement funding was coming from. There are many possible reasons that nurses who are of retirement age are choosing not to retire.

For whatever reason, however, more and more nurses are choosing not to retire and thus contribute to the flood of nurses in certain areas. Sadly, this will continue for many more years since housing prices are not predicted to increase or return to the 2005 levels for many, many years.

You see, we do not live in a current economic market that is conducive to newly graduated RNs who want to obtain experience in the hospital systems, which is the place that most nursing programs are grooming their nurses to work in. Hospitals spend a lot of money on their experienced nursing staff, but the staff is not ready to – or is choosing not to – retire, given today's economic uncertainties. This means that some nurses of retirement age are holding on to positions that newly graduated nurses need.

Are you in a flooded market?

In order to land your first RN position, we need to know, are you in a flooded area? How challenging will it be for you to land this first job? So, how do you find out if you are in a flooded area or not? Hop on the internet! I love using Indeed.com as my go-to job search engine. Indeed.com pulls from Monster.com, CareerBuilder.com, iHispano.com and many other websites so it is a one-stop shop, which is why I love it.

Let's start with a simple search for a "nurse" position, but let's compare a couple of states as of April 1, 2012. First, we will search the current outlook of certain states. For this example, I will pick Illinois and Florida to compare. In the "what" field on www.Indeed.com, type in "nurse." Then in the "where" field, put in "IL." Next, repeat your search in the same way, but use "FL" for Florida in this case.

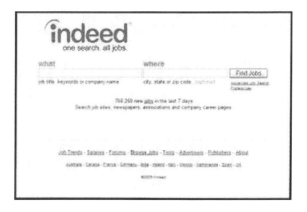

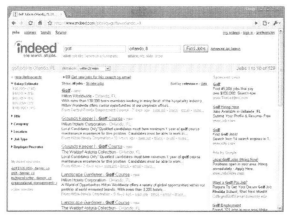

Now look at the left-hand side of the screen under "Salary Estimate," and you will see that in Illinois there are 9,441 positions for nurses at a $30,000-income level. I am not saying to focus on a $30K position. Rather, I am teaching you how to look at and think about the statistics that are here in front of you. Likely, the $30,000 positions are for Licensed Practical Nurses, LPNs, but using the keyword "nurse" will still include these in your search return. Interesting. Next, look at Florida; there are 19,642 positions. Clearly, there is more of a nursing shortage in Florida, thus creating a higher demand for nurses there.

ILLINOIS:

Salary Estimate

$30,000+ (9441)
$50,000+ (7271)
$70,000+ (4533)
$90,000+ (1837)
$110,000+ (806)

FLORIDA:

Salary Estimate

$30,000+ (19642)
$50,000+ (15862)
$70,000+ (6256)
$90,000+ (2627)
$110,000+ (1412)

Now let's do some more digging... Change your key words. We will still compare Illinois to Florida, but this time, type in "new graduate nurse" in the appropriate field. You should see:

ILLINOIS:

Salary Estimate

$40,000+ (468)
$60,000+ (362)
$80,000+ (178)

$100,000+ (63)

$120,000+ (34)

FLORIDA:

Salary Estimate

$40,000+ (1528)

$60,000+ (1152)

$80,000+ (338)

$100,000+ (187)

$120,000+ (153)

Look at the positions that are being offered in each area. In the shortage areas (i.e., the *non*-flooded areas), you will easily find specialty positions waiting for you with open arms! What do I mean by specialty positions? ER/ED, ICU, OB, etc. This does *not* include medical/surgical.

If you are in a flooded area, however, you should be thrilled to take any hospital position that will give you a chance to gain the needed experience that makes you appealing to employers. Again, your goal with your first RN position is to gain the magical amount of 1 to 2 years worth of experience, so you can bounce into a higher-paying position after that timeframe, as we have previously discussed.

> **"You have to see every potential roadblock as an opportunity and a benefit."**
>
> -- Suze Orman

If you must stay

If you absolutely cannot move and you are in a flooded market there is still hope. First of all, you need to apply to every position that is available. Full-time income may be the goal, but a full-time position may be hard to come by. Take anything. Think about how any position will impact your resume. On a resume, it does not say "I worked 30 hours a week for 12 months at ABC Hospital."

Instead, you list the amount of time in months and years that you have been at a position. Again, do not get wrapped around the axel about this first position. The experience is the important part. If you cannot move out of a flooded market and cannot obtain gainful employment at a hospital, you need to search other avenues ASAP.

Remember, the ticking time bomb of paying back your student loans and the accruing interest, as well the ticking time bomb of needing to amass 1 to 2 years of experience have started. Right now, you simply need to get into the game. I encourage you to have a bigger vision and look at the bigger picture of your long-term nursing career when applying for nursing jobs.

Skilled nursing facilities

Look at SNFs, skilled nursing facilities, aka LTC/long-term care. This would be my second choice (after the hospital) to gain experience because of the bright future that it can offer. Having SNF experience will open *many* doors to you.

Think about it, the baby-boom generation, the largest percentage of people in America, will be utilizing the SNF market in the very near future. The hospital is no longer a place for people to recuperate from illness or surgery. Rather, people are discharged to the rehabilitation wing of an SNF to recoup.

Insurance industry

Another area that you can look at is the insurance industry. Let me guess, this is not "real" nursing to you? Consider this, it is a *real* RN job, and your loan payments are starting! From here, you can bounce into case management, risk management or possibly a higher level of management. Those positions do not require you to be on call; they do not require you to work weekends or holidays, and they pay through the roof! Is that real enough for you?

If you have only been presented with bedside nursing as the pinnacle of your RN career, I could see how you would feel that these are not "real" nursing positions. I do not feel that bedside nursing is the pinnacle of your career. I encourage you to think bigger, much bigger.

Also, it is important to note that all clinical nurses must keep their skills current. For example, in the not-so-long-ago past, IVs were not initiated with retractable needle devices. So, if a clinical nurse had 25 years of hands-on experience, stepped away for 18 months and then returned to nursing, she/he would now have to perfect her/his skill of starting IVs, utilizing this newer device.

With that being said, if as a nurse you were never afforded the opportunity to learn certain hands-on skill sets such as starting IVs, why wouldn't you take a non-clinical RN position so that you can utilize your nursing thought process, rationales, critical thinking, etc.?

You can function as an RN in either a clinical or a non-clinical role. You can impact lives in either fashion. The imminent goal is to help you land a position, be it in a clinical or a non-clinical role!

Correctional facilities

The next area that I highly suggest you look at is within correctional facilities. Take a deep breath here because you may panic at this recommendation before you fully understand the rationale.

First of all, I have personally worked in a state maximum security prison, and, wow, I learned a ton! It is interesting to me, being in the Chicago-land market especially, that RNs do not think twice about working in the ER/ED but raise an eyebrow at the correctional facilities.

Think about it...In the ER/ED, you could be caring for a gang member who just got hit in crossfire from a rival gang. The security personnel at the hospital are your only line of defense *when* the rival gang members enter the ER/ED to finish the attack! Security only has a walkie-talkie to defend you – no weapon. Not to mention that an ER/ED nurse must pay particular attention to the level of customer service that he or she is delivering at all times – even when dealing with a gang banger! So if the gang banger reports that you were not this, that and a bag of chips, *your* income could suffer. REALLY? Yes. Does anyone else see a problem here?

In the correctional facility, the only weapons are with the guards, not with the inmates. Should an issue arise in the infirmary (i.e., the ER within the correctional facility), the guards have your back. The medical personnel in a correction facility are treated like Switzerland; they are seen as neutral ground. The inmates are grateful if you are simply passionate about the care you give them. And you are always passionate about the care that you give! That is part of being a nurse!

In addition, the experience that you can gain at a correctional facility is multifaceted. If you are at a female prison, you have a chance to gain experience in medical/surgical, surgical post op, psych, cardiac/telemetry, dialysis, minute clinic and OB.

Working for a system

Here is a true story. "Jess" was a bachelor-degree-seeking student nurse of mine who graduated December of 2008. Like so many, she could not find a position as an RN, so she continued to work as a Certified Nursing Assistant (CNA). How depressing not to land an RN position – not to mention continuing to work and get paid as a CNA – after all that schooling! She worked *so* hard in school, passed boards on the first try and no one would hire her because she did not have any experience as an RN. Now mind you, she had over two years of experience as a CNA in a SNF and in hospice!

Anyway, Jess was not able to move out of the area, and she was quickly feeling defeated. Finally, in June of 2009, she reached out for help. After a long conversation, I suggested that she apply to Wexford, an internal staffing company for the prison system. She secured a position as an RN and started in July of 2009.

After a mere four months of working at the prison, Jess picked up a full-time position as an office nurse within a healthcare system. That is key: she did not work for a specific medical doctor (MD) or doctor of Osteopathic Medicine (DO), but rather, she worked for a hospital *system*.

Interestingly, Jess came in at the *top* of the office pay scale because she had such a vast array of experience! That is right: she maxed out the pay scale, even though she only had a few *months* of experience as an RN! Are you starting to think differently now? Remember, this is not about finding a position for you to keep forever throughout your entire nursing career, but rather, it is a strategic stepping stone in your career!

Jess's ultimate nursing career goal was not to work as a corrections nurse. Now, there is nothing wrong with that goal, it just was not *her* goal. Jess's ultimate goal was to work at a hospital, and she continued to work toward that goal.

As time passed, "Jess" juggled the two positions, working part time at the prison as needed, to enhance her income and to show that she worked at that position for a longer period of time, which is another technique to help land a competitive RN position! But, Jess knew what her goal was, which was to work at a hospital. And now that Jess was already working for the health system, she was considered an internal candidate when a pediatric/medical surgical RN position became open at the hospital. Additionally, she had been working with various MDs/DOs at the office who helped her with references!

Guess what? Jess now works full time at the hospital as a pediatric/medical surgical RN, which is what she wanted to do! More than likely, her pay is higher than others who had have started there straight out of school. The best part is that Jess has been an RN since 2009, but her experience base is broad, which will help her immensely in her future RN career.

Jess was up for the challenge. Will you be? Jess became successful. Will you become successful? Jess is as good as or better than those who came before her. Will you be?

In order to succeed, you must build your *knowledge*, take *action* and overcome your *fear*. You must take the knowledge that I have given you – about flooded nursing markets – and combine that with action to gain the experience you need to land your ultimate nursing job.

Now you know how to tell if you are in a flooded market or not, as well as how to gain nursing experience in a flooded market. In the following chapter, we will discuss the pros and cons of taking a full-time versus part-time nursing position.

> **"If you are not willing to risk the unusual, you will have to settle for the ordinary."**
>
> -- Jim Rohn

Chapter 7:

Full Time vs. Part Time

When you are ready to make a choice, how do you know what position to apply for or which position to accept? I know, I know, this sort of information is never covered in nursing school!

However, maximizing your time and increasing your monetary compensation is an important component of nursing – it's *huge*! And so is keeping your sanity by not working, working, working until you drop! But I am here to show you that there is a way to maximize your time and money while working reasonable hours and keeping your sanity! In order to achieve this balance, though, it is *vital* that you follow my guidance regarding your nursing professional career. So, let's dive right in and talk about *what* type of positions to take, and more importantly, *why* you should take them.

Thus, the question becomes, should you accept full-time or part-time work? Believe it or not, you may not want a full-time position after you learn this next technique! Remember that your goal is to maximize your income – and not work to death while doing it!

Some of you may not know the lingo of RN employment, so let's start there. A full-time, 40-hour-a-week position is considered a 1.0 position, based on 8-hour shifts. This can also be done for 12-hour shifts; however, this example will focus on 8-hour shifts.

Pay periods

Let's look at the calendar below, focusing on the first two weeks of the month, the first pay period:

SUN	MON	TUE	WED	THU	FRI	SAT
1	2 X	3 X	4 X	5 X	6 X	7
8	9 X	10 X	11 X	12 X	13 X	14
15	16	17	18	19	20	21
22	23	24	25	26	27	28
29	30	31				

If we assume that you have the normal weekend period (i.e., Saturday and Sunday) off and that you work a 1.0 position, you would work 10 of the 14 days in a pay period. Again, looking at the calendar above, do you see which 10 days I am talking about?

Now, if you work a 0.8 position, it is possible that you are still considered a full-time employee, since each hospital has different guidelines regarding what constitutes full-time status. However, the important point here is that with a 0.8 position, you would only work four days each week, or eight days of the pay period (see calendar below). In this example, do you see which eight days you would work?

SUN	MON	TUE	WED	THU	FRI	SAT
1	2 X	3 X	4 X	5 X	6	7
8	9 X	10 X	11 X	12 X	13	14
15	16	17	18	19	20	21
22	23	24	25	26	27	28
29	30	31				

This can also be done if you have a 0.5 position, as well (see calendar below). However, a 0.5 position is definitely considered part-time status.

SUN	MON	TUE	WED	THU	FRI	SAT
1	2	3 X	4 X	5 X	6	7
8	9	10 X	11 X	12	13	14
15	16	17	18	19	20	21
22	23	24	25	26	27	28
29	30	31				

With this example, do you see the five days that you would work in this pay period?

Please note that the examples provided are merely visual representations of sample schedules, so that you can easily visualize the different scenarios. I am not saying that you will have all weekends off or will always work the first three days of a pay period or whatever. On the contrary, in nursing, your schedule will *fluctuate* immensely! However, I hope that these scheduling examples help to demonstrate the different ways in which nurses are classified as full-time or part-time employees.

Drawbacks of a 1.0 position

I do not necessarily recommend taking a 1.0 (full-time) position. Why not? Simple. The majority of staff nursing positions require nurses to be on-call from time to time in addition to working their normal hours as determined by their point status.

Let me give you an example of how this might work. Let's say that a nurse in the emergency department (ED) accepts a 1.0, full-time-equivalent (FTE) position. In addition to her or his 1.0, 40-hour-per-week position, this nurse will be required to pick up on-call hours as normal customary practice. This means that even if the nurse is off-duty, she or he must report to her or his unit within 30 minutes of being called or notified if help is needed. Did you catch that? These are extra hours that are mandated over time but are only called for when a unit census dictates necessity.

This may not sound like a big deal, but if you are already working 40 hours a week, *when* will you feel like coming into work and putting in additional hours if you have to? Remember, this is a common practice in many healthcare organizations and is therefore a requirement of many hospital or medical units. It is also important to remember that if a unit is short-staffed to begin with, there is a very high likelihood that you *will* be called in to work when you are on call.

However, *if* you work a 0.8 position, you have more options as to when you are available to be on call!

Also, keep in mind that you should create your financial budget around the amount of pay that you expect to receive based *only* on your FTE status, whether it is 1.0, 0.8, or 0.5. This is because you cannot count on receiving constant pay for on-call duty since the unit's need for this may fluctuate. However, know that while you are only paid a small amount to be available for on-call status, you will usually receive monetary compensation at a rate of time-and-a-half for the hours that you are actually called in to work an on-call status.

Flex hours

Another thing to keep in mind as you choose an FTE status and create your financial budget is that a hospital will "flex" employees' hours up or down based on need, meaning that a hospital may send employees home or cut down their hours when the census in the unit is slow. What I am saying is that you should not necessarily count on a full-time paycheck each pay period, since a nursing position does not necessarily guarantee job or income stability.

Gaining more hours

Next, I would like to demonstrate a technique that several of my students have incorporated in order to gain more hours and thus increase their pay. First, they accept a FTE position of 0.8 or less. Then, after orientation at the hospital or healthcare organization, they ask other RNs if they would like a day off. If the RNs ask why, my students simply respond that they are looking to pick up more hours. Usually, this is easily accomplished! In this fashion, the new nurses find themselves working more hours than a 0.8 position calls for!

But remember that with this technique, hours are not guaranteed. However, hours may not be guaranteed even if these nurses sign up for a 1.0-FTE position, since again, the hospital can flex hours up or down if a unit's census is low. So be sure not to get lulled into a false sense of job security!

I recommend that after six months have passed, the "experienced" new nurse should pick up additional registry, Quinn or temp-in-house hours at another hospital *instead* of picking up extra hours at the first hospital. This is because these positions typically pay *more* per hour because they do not come with benefits. Also, in addition to increasing pay, this technique affords you more experience! Furthermore, you now have more security or stability in the case of hospital downsizing, since you are splitting your hours between two hospitals!

Remember that you need to build your base wide and strong so that when something unexpected happens, you are prepared! Another way that this technique will help you build a strong base is to provide you with a bigger network of people to draw from when you are ready to take on greater nursing roles and responsibilities. With this technique, you learn from more than one hospital and are able to demonstrate to potential employers that you are skilled at juggling responsibilities and managing multiple schedules! Win!

Check the benefits

Now, let's talk about employer-offered benefits, such as group medical insurance. If you think that you need to work full time simply to get benefits, stop. First, check with the organization's HR department to see if the employer offers benefits for part-time workers. Some organizations offer benefits to part-time employees, but at a greater out-of-pocket cost to the employee. Let's run some numbers as an example.

Pretend that an organization offers full-time benefits for an employee and the employee's family at a cost of $300.00 a month. The organization also offers the same benefits for part-time employees and their families, but at a cost of $600.00 a month. Given this scenario, most people would jump at the full-time position.

But hmm, let's think this over! Let's say that you took a part-time position as well as picked up an additional position, say a registry, Quinn or temp-in-house position, at another hospital. In that case, you would make more money hourly, which would *easily* make up the difference in the prices of benefits. (Also, remember that neither a full-time nor a part-time position will guarantee that you are not flexed from your hours. Thus, you cannot say that working a 1.0-FTE position at one hospital is more financially stable than working multiple 0.5 positions at two hospitals. Both hospitals will flex the staff's hours when unit census is low.)

1.0 vs. FTE jobs

Mariah works a 1.0 FTE at Hospital ABC and pays $300.00 a month to receive benefits. She is hired at a pay rate of $25.00 an hour, working 40 hours a week, which equals pay of $1,000 a week.

Before taxes, she earns $4,000 a month. If we subtract $300 for benefit costs, we see that Mariah receives $3,700 in pay per month before taxes.

Instead of working a 1.0 FTE, Mariah works a 0.5 FTE at Hospital ABC and pays $600.00 a month to receive benefits. She is hired at a pay rate of $25.00 an hour and works 20 hours per week. Here, Mariah makes $2,000 a month. If we subtract $600 for benefit costs, we see that Mariah receives $1,400 in pay per month before taxes.

But, in this second example, Mariah additionally works a registry, Quinn or temp-in-house position at another hospital. This gig pays her $30.00 an hour. Mariah works here for 20 hours every week, and she makes $2,400 a month before taxes. Therefore, this scenario gives Mariah a total of $3,800 a month in pay before taxes for working at two different hospitals. Mariah is making *an extra* $100.00 and has the option of working fewer hours to bring home the same amount of money that she would have in the first scenario!

So, if you have only one option, which is to accept a part-time position, *jump on it!* You may still come out on top. Of course, if you have the options to accept either a full-time or a part-time position, you should weigh the options and choose what's best for you. But as you make your choice, do not fall victim to the myth that you need to work full-time to receive full benefits! If the part-time benefits cost more, but you are being paid more (or are working less for the same amount of money), it may be more beneficial for you to take two part-time positions instead of one full-time position.

Outside the hospital

Here is something else for you to ponder: Another positive reason to accept a part-time position is that it allows you to be flexible and thus open to additional nursing opportunities.

Remember when I said that nursing schools primarily direct your associations with nursing toward the clinical aspects, such as working at a hospital, long-term-care facility, or doctor's office? Well, this focus may preclude you from thinking about nursing in a way that's outside the box. What do I mean by this?

Well, if you take a 1.0 position at a hospital or other facility, then your schedule will be too busy to allow you to accept alternative nursing positions, which may appeal to those nurses who are looking for something other than typical RN roles.

Additionally, when you have a 1.0 position, you may fall into the false sense of security of having a stable income with no surprises. But instead of following the comfortable route, the one that is touted by the majority of nursing programs, I greatly encourage you to be *uncomfortable*, so that you self-motivate to reach for a bigger vision than the one that is spoon-fed to you at nursing school.

Knowledge and action

You can rise to any occasion and accomplish more than what has previously been presented to you. The opportunities are truly limitless – you simply need someone to show you the way!

In order to succeed, you must build your *knowledge*, take *action* and overcome your *fear*. You must take the knowledge that I have given you – the benefits of accepting a part-time nursing position – and combine that with action to land your dream job!

In this chapter, I hope I have taught you to look at assumptions about nursing in a different light and think outside the box when it comes to choosing between accepting a full-time and part-time nursing position. In the following chapter, we will explore additional assumptions about the different types of nursing so that you can begin to think creatively about nursing specialties, as well.

> "Here's to the crazy ones, the misfits, the rebels, the troublemakers, the round pegs in the square holes ... the ones who see things differently -- they're not fond of rules, and they have no respect for the status quo... You can quote them, disagree with them, glorify or vilify them, but the only thing you can't do is ignore them because they change things... They push the human race forward, and while some may see them as the crazy ones, we see genius, because the people who are crazy enough to think that they can change the world, are the ones who do."
>
> -- Steve Jobs

Chapter 8:

What Type of Nursing?

When I graduated from nursing school, I knew that I wanted to work in the Labor and Delivery, L&D, unit. I was passionate about it merely from what I experienced during my nursing clinical rotation. A vast majority of my nursing instructors, however, told me that I should not and could not go straight into a specialty unit. They said that, instead, I first needed to work on a medical/surgical (or med/surg, as it's commonly known) floor.

That was gut-wrenching news to me. I despised my med/surg rotations in school, just like many of you may despise L&D. (But it is all good; not everyone will love every area, so do not worry! If we all enjoyed the same type of nursing, then that would *really* cause "issues" in the job market!) I did not understand why I was being told that I needed to work in med/surg first. Was it because these instructors did not go into a specialty position as their first career move, and they wanted me to emulate what they had done? All of a sudden, I started to question what others took as fact. I started to think outside the box about nursing.

Path less taken

In order to better understand why certain instructors or managers say what they say, let's examine this matter from the nurse manager's perspective. Let's pretend that I did go into med/surg first. Let's say that after one year on the med/surg floor, I became an amazing med/surg staff RN who by that time knew the ropes of the unit.

In this case, *why* would my nurse manager want to let me go? What incentive would she have to recommend me to the L&D nurse manager, either at that same institution or elsewhere?

Would I have any L&D specialty skills after working for one year on the med/surg floor? No. Other than teaching me how to start IVs or helping me learn certain skills such as time management or other pertinent skills that might set me apart from the others who are clamoring for an L&D position, how would my time on the med/surg floor enable me to excel and set myself apart from the rest of the pack? It would not.

Now, let's pretend that I chose to go straight into L&D after nursing school. Think like the nurse manager again. As a newly graduated RN, I could be molded to the L&D mindset from the onset. This is important from a nurse manager's perspective because it means that I do not need to break any bad habits I may have been exposed to in a different specialty unit. I would also be quite eager to learn and excel, and not have any signs or symptoms of burn-out.

Which path did I choose? You guessed right: I took the path less taken. I did not listen to the instructors, and I applied exclusively for L&D positions. However, by doing so, I ran into a challenge that some of you might face. The challenge was that any open nursing positions that were located close to my home – positions in Level II L&D units in the southwest suburbs of Chicago – would not take me because I did not have experience. Sound familiar? However, I was determined to land a nursing position in an L&D unit, so I increased my search area to include more possible health organizations in which I would be willing to work.

> "Your time is limited, so don't waste it living someone else's life. Don't be trapped by dogma - which is living with the results of other people's thinking. Don't let the noise of other's opinions drown out your own inner voice. And most important, have the courage to follow your heart and intuition. They somehow already know what you truly want to become. Everything else is secondary."
>
> -- Steve Jobs

You're hired!

It ended up that I accepted a position just off Lake Shore Drive, in the northern portion of Chicago. Without traffic, my commute to work was just more than an hour each way. This was not ideal or the way I had pictured things going after graduation, but I had done it: I had landed an L&D position straight out of nursing school and was working three 12-hour shifts a week from 7 pm to 7 am on my assigned days.

And guess what? I never worked that shift. Why? Orientation on a specialty unit last three or more months. And I had just finished my orientation when it became time for me to be an L&D patient!

That is correct; at the end of my L&D orientation, I was due with our first child. Of course, I had not mentioned my pregnancy at the job interview! Unlike the women in the previous generations of my family, I needed to work full time.

At one point during my pregnancy, I was finally offered a position that was closer to home and offered better pay, so I jumped at the opportunity!

How did I come across this opportunity? You see, I went to my local hospital for the birth of our first child, and during the admission process, the RN asked if I had taken any child-birth classes. When I honestly answered, "No," she just looked at me and smiled. Then she asked me what my background was because it sounded to her like I knew more than the average person about L&D. Of course at that point I told her that I was an L&D RN!

She lit up like a Christmas tree and told me that they were short staffed. She asked me if I would ever consider applying – for real! Certainly, I was excited, but I needed to tell her that I did not have a year of experience yet. It turns out that she did not care since I had *some* experience and they were short staffed!

I kid you not; the Women's Health Nurse Manager interviewed me for the position on *postpartum*. I started six weeks later, in an L&D unit that was close to home – and they offered me a bit of a pay raise, too! *Yeah*!

> "Life is too short to not pursue your dreams. Someday your life will near its end and all you will be able to do is look backwards. You can reflect with joy or regret. Those who dream, who set goals and act on them to live out their dreams are those who live lives of joy and have a

> sense of peace when they near the end of their lives. They have finished well, for themselves and for their families."
>
> -- Jim Rohn

Your initial goal

Once you graduate from nursing school, I recommend that you make it your initial goal to gain *experience* by whatever legitimate means necessary. Take whatever positions you can to obtain the needed 12 to 24 months or more of experience that employers are looking for. *But*, you should also have your *next* position in mind.

Thinking about your next desired position will help you realize what type of experience it is that you should be focused on obtaining right now.

Once you have read through the alternative nursing opportunities that I will present to you in a subsequent chapter and have gained perspective about the bigger vision of nursing, I urge you to do some research *immediately*. Look at the positions that you are interested in obtaining, and find out how much and what type of experience the positions call for. Then I recommend that you look at *all* the positions you have chosen, and make a decision about which type of nursing you would like to pursue, based solely on your own needs and desires.

No cookie-cutter mold

Not every employer will require experience in a specialty unit like mine did. And not every employer will require general medical-floor experience either. Simply put, there just isn't a cookie-cutter mold for RNs to follow when deciding which path to pursue. Period.

Remember to ask yourself, as I did, "Will I be up to the challenge? Will I become successful? Will I be as good as or better than those who came before me?" In order to succeed, you must build your *knowledge*, take *action,* and overcome your *fear*. You must take the knowledge that I have given you – the perspective to question the status quo and make decisions based on your own desires for your nursing career – and combine that with action to land your dream job!

In this chapter, I hope that I have taught you to look at assumptions about nursing in a different light and think outside the box when it comes to choosing a nursing specialty or path to pursue. In the next chapter, we will explore alternative nursing options regarding location, types of facilities in which to work, and avenues through which to find your dream nursing job!

Chapter 9:

Your Next Job

The nursing profession offers *unlimited* career possibilities. Yet, sadly, most nursing professionals do not know how to venture beyond the stereotypical roles of nursing. But get ready, because I see a vision that reaches *far* beyond the norm, and I will guide you in a step-by-step fashion to show you how to achieve your goal!

Now the question is, what types of nursing roles are you willing to fill and where are you willing to go to do it? I am here to show you the possibilities. I am here to show you *how* to think differently and how to advance your career by doing so.

Debt or degree

"CeCe" is a single mother who lives in a rural farm town that is located an hour and 20 minutes outside and southwest of Chicago. She is 51 years old, and in 2011 when we first met, she had recently finished her Master's of Science degree in Nursing. CeCe's RN experience had been exclusively at one facility, an outpatient surgical facility in a nearby town. After finishing her

MSN, she fully intended to utilize her advanced degree and was interested in teaching at the university level.

Similar to many others, CeCe had incurred a significant amount of student-loan debt as she was obtaining her MSN. Thus, CeCe began to realize that the surgical facility that she was working at was not an area which would further her career. And after having worked so hard for her MSN, CeCe wanted to utilize it!

Hence, I met CeCe at the university where I taught. The university would not hire her full time because they were short of and needed to hire RNs with post-graduate degrees, such as PhDs, DNPs, EDDs, etc. For the sake of the university's scholastic reputation, they need to staff a certain percentage of the faculty with post-graduate-degree members. Thus, they could not hire CeCe with only her MSN.

In other words, in order for CeCe to become a full-time faculty member, she would need to return to post-graduate school full time for three to four years and incur $60,000 or more in student-loan debt in the hope that there would be a position available for her at the time that she finally finished her post-graduate work.

This was a bit of a wake-up call for CeCe. She had left the outpatient surgical facility thinking that she would easily land a full-time teaching position now that she had an MSN. Not so. Fortunately, CeCe was easily able to secure multiple adjunct (i.e., part-time) teaching positions, but nothing full time. Unfortunately, this is a common scenario in the education industry, even when so-called authorities are touting that there is a dramatic shortage of nursing instructors. This sounds similar to direct-entry staff nursing, now doesn't it?

Teaching jobs

The business sector of all colleges and universities knows that it is in their best interest to hire many part-time, adjunct instructors instead of hiring full-time instructors without post-graduate degrees because the part-time instructors may not be eligible to receive full-time benefits, such as healthcare or 401(k) benefits (NEA Higher Education Advocate, Vol. 29, No. 2, March 2012). You should keep in mind that this is not something that is exclusive to the nursing or education industries. This is a growing trend that occurs throughout our entire economy.

> **"Find someone who is willing to share the truth with you."**
>
> -- Jim Rohn

Think like a businessperson

Because of these types of financial challenges that face both the nursing industry and general economy these days, I urge each and every one of you to build your base strong and wide. You need to think like a businessperson in nursing now.

In order to illustrate this point, allow us to examine possible employment scenarios that would benefit CeCe. For instance, I received the following notice of available nursing positions from a recruiter, and I immediately thought of CeCe.

Possible nursing positions for CeCe

Carmen Kosicek,

Would you like to pay off your student loans while working with the Alaska Native population? We have already placed 8 Registered Nurses in these positions over the past year and they love it! Please review the information below and call me today at (214) 442-XXXX if you are qualified and interested in any of the positions below. I am very excited to tell you all about the positions and the area! Positions include ER, Med/Surg, Operating Room, and Labor and Delivery.

Position #57868

* Job: ER Staff Position

* Shifts: Varied 12 Hour Shifts Available

* Pay: $38.92 per Hour

* Student Loans: $20K Paid Each Year for 3 Years

* Bonus: 7-8% of Your Annual Salary Each Year ($5,666 - $6,476)

* Qualifications: 2-3 Years Working in an ER Setting Required

Position #57837

* Job: Inpatient Med / Surg

* Shifts: Varied 12 Hour Shifts Available

* Pay: $38.92 per Hour

* Student Loans: $20K Paid Each Year for 3 Years

* Bonus: 7-8% of Your Annual Salary Each Year ($5,666 - $6,476)

* Qualifications: 2-3 Years Working in a Hospital Med / Surg * Setting With Both Adults and Children Required

Position #57838

* Job: Operating Room Staff Position

* Shifts: Monday Friday Day Shift

* Pay: $38.92 per Hour

* Student Loans: $20K Paid Each Year for 3 Years

* Bonus: 7-8% of Your Annual Salary Each Year ($5,666 - $6,476)

* Qualifications: 2-3 Years Working in an Operating Room With * Both Scrubbing and Circulating Required

Position #52193

* Job: Labor and Delivery Staff Position

* Shifts: Varied 12 Hour Shifts Available

* Pay: $38.92 per Hour

* Student Loans: $20K Paid Each Year for 3 Years

* Bonus: 7-8% of Your Annual Salary Each Year ($5,666 - $6,476)

* Qualifications: 2-3 Years Working in Labor and Delivery With Newborn, Post-Partum, and Delivery

Other Benefits for Each Position:

* 23 Days of Paid Time Off PLUS 10 Paid Holidays

* Medical, Dental, Vision

* Retirement Program With Company Match

* $12,500 Relocation Paid for by the Facility

* 30 Days of Free Housing to Find a Place to Live

Location for All FOUR Positions:

* Help an Underserved Alaskan Community and Their Loved Ones in this Remote Setting

* 8% Higher Salaries Than the National Average Paid by this Large Hospital System

* See Native American Eskimo Population and Become a Part of Their Culture

* King Salmon Fishing, Big Game Hunting, Kayaking, and Boating Await You

* Multiple Restaurants, Local College, and Regional Airport With Multiple Daily Direct Flights to Anchorage

* Must Be Comfortable Living in a Rural Location - Not Anchorage, Juneau, or Fairbanks

Sincerely,

Ray |Recruiting Team Lead

(866) 633-xxxx x4807 | (214) 442-xxxx (direct) | (215) 243-xxxx (fax)

XXXXX Healthcare Placement | Rxxxx@xxxcp.com

Benefit of taking the position

Why do I think that taking a nursing position with Native Americans in Alaska would be a great business move for CeCe? Well, one of the great things about working in Alaska is that CeCe would avoid paying state income taxes! Being that CeCe is in her 50s, she should realize that by taking one these available positions, she could additionally completely wipe out her student-loan debt!

In contrast, if CeCe takes a position elsewhere, she would have to pay state income taxes on the amount of money she makes before she can put that money toward paying down her student loans. In this manner, it would take CeCe a long time to pay off her student-loan debt, especially as she only has a single income.

Also, in most cases, student-loan debt is not something that you can include in a bankruptcy. Student-loan debt usually stays with you for life. Let's say that CeCe does not want to move to Alaska to take advantage of this smart business opportunity. If she chooses to stay where she is, it is probable that she may never be able to retire. Why, you ask? Think about it this way: If CeCe first pays state income taxes then pays her bills and living expenses then pays down a certain amount of her student loans, how much can she really put away for retirement?

Now, let's also look at this scenario from another – non-business-oriented – perspective. Let's look at it from the point of view of what is best for CeCe's family. CeCe's youngest child will be entering high school in fall of 2012. Before her daughter starts a new school, CeCe might want to embrace the Alaskan opportunity while it is easier for her daughter to make the move with her. Given that CeCe and her family's relocation would be paid for (as outlined in the job postings above), now would be a great time for them to head out on an amazing adventure. And as a parent, CeCe can be comforted by knowing that the hospital and school systems in Alaska are of the same climate as anywhere else in America!

My point with CeCe's story is that there are many ways to look at a situation, but it is important to approach a situation from the vantage point of what it can offer you. If CeCe chooses to move to Alaska, in three short years she could come out with no student-loan debt, wonderful adventures, an amazing life story, and money in the bank for her future.

Even if CeCe does not think that this particular opportunity is right for her and her family, she should be proactive and reach out to the recruiter. Perhaps the recruiter knows of other openings in other underserved areas of the country. In this way, CeCe can uncover the possibilities that could be right in front of her without her even knowing it. Now, this is thinking like a businessperson, a networker.

There may be many reasons that CeCe would choose not to take a position like this, all of which are valid for her personal situation. My aim in examining the above scenarios is simply to demonstrate how many opportunities exist that you may not be aware of. And know that not all available positions will take you to Alaska, but then again, some people would love a chance to have an Alaskan adventure! And heck, think of it this way, Chicago gets a lot of cold weather, snow, and ice, similar to cities in Alaska, and the opportunities in Chicago right now may not compete with those in Alaska!

Think big

I agree that logistically speaking, not everyone can move to certain areas of the country. But beyond making a specific geographic move, what I do encourage you to do is think *big* enough to recognize the opportunities that are presented in your life. How will you see an opportunity in front of you if you do not know what to look for?

> "You don't have to see the whole staircase, just take the First Step."
>
> -- Dr. Martin Luther King

Go hunting

If you already have your bachelor's degree, then let's start your *hunt*! Stop right there. Notice that I said bachelor's degree. Did you notice that I did not say specifically say a Bachelor of Science in Nursing (BSN)?

That is because there may be those of you out there who already have a bachelor's degree in specializations other than nursing but who have returned to school to get an RN certification. If this applies to you and you already have a BA or BS, then you may want to think about a couple of things, as I will explain directly below.

Number one: In order to advance upwardly within a hospital setting, you will need to have at least a BSN. Both the Magnet Status and Nursing 2020 Vision are proof of this. Remember, though, that this information is only relevant if you plan to spend the duration of your nursing career at a hospital. However, I will show you how to find RN positions outside the hospital that pay more, have more positions available for you to choose from and call only for a BA or BS degree rather than a specific BSN.

Number two: You may be wondering which educational path to choose to obtain your RN certification if you already have a BA or BS and are accepted to both an ADN (associate degree in nursing) program as well as a BSN program? Well, either way, it will take you two or more years to complete each of these programs. So now you need to factor both the out-of-pocket expense of obtaining your RN certification and your age into your thought process and future plans for nursing.

Cost/benefit analysis

Do you really need another piece of paper – a degree certificate – to advance your nursing career? Weigh out the cost versus the benefits for each scenario. Also, remember what I told you earlier: if your goal is to stay in a hospital setting or other traditional RN environment, such as a long-term care facility, doctor's office or teaching environment, then yes, you must have at least a BSN.

However, if you already have a piece of paper, a BA or BS in another specialty, you can still make more income *if* you look to less-traditional nursing environments. And again, in these less-traditional arenas, there are a larger variety of nursing roles and a larger number of available positions, and more often than not, you simply need just *one* BA or BS, as well as an active RN license, to succeed.

Let me also add that I am not a big fan of career-bedside staff nursing. No, there is nothing wrong with this type of nursing, but I have to ask: If you already have a BA or BS, why not utilize it to its fullest potential? Why continue to work holidays and weekends and for less pay at a bedside nursing position when you are more financially valuable than that? Why work under such physically demanding conditions if there is a different way for you to succeed in nursing?

Multiple degrees

"Roz", a nursing student of mine, already had *two* bachelor's degrees when I met her. This is because her initial intent was to become a lawyer. She had a BA in Political Science, and a BS in Business Management. Roz also already had thousands of dollars in student-loan debt. Sadly, her two degrees had not helped her achieve gainful and financially stable employment.

Thus, Roz returned to college to get an RN degree, and she chose to pursue another bachelor's degree as the means by which to get her RN degree. Roz had not been shown another way. She believed, correctly, that it would take her two years to become an RN. However, she incorrectly surmised that, given the time it would take to earn her RN, it would be in her best interest to pursue a BSN, as well.

Why had Roz followed the traditional route and spent so much time getting multiple bachelor's degrees to become an RN? Well, one explanation is that Roz comes from a family of nurses. Roz told me that nursing is a respected profession in her Filipino culture. I can see why that is, considering that nursing is a respected profession across the globe. And, after all, RNs typically get a decent hourly wage and are known to be hard-working.

Roz's mother was an RN for nearly 30 years. However, Roz's mother did not encourage Roz to become an RN, even though most of the women in the family were RNs. I asked why. Roz said that her mother had told her that being an RN was physically demanding. This is true – if you spend your nursing career at the bedside, which Roz's mother did.

Roz then told me that she did not see herself being an RN in a hospital setting for more than 3 to 4 years. This is because she remembers how exhausted her mother was after working her shifts, especially as she became older.

Although I was excited to hear that Roz was open to nursing ventures outside the typical hospital bedside setting, sadly, Roz did not know what else she could do with the RN degree that she had already spent so much time and money pursuing. Roz had a singular vision and assumed that she would be an Advanced-Practice Nurse in the future ... until I showed Roz all the options available to her!!

Roz's husband's story

Then I asked Roz about her husband. Here is her husband's story.

"Tim" has his BS and went straight from school to working in a medical-device production line for about 3 to 4 years. He worked with engineers; although he was not an engineer himself. His second job was as a medical-device production-line supervisor, and he worked in that role for just less than one year. Then, for the next five to six years, Tim worked with a consulting company as a validation engineer. And now, at his fourth job, which he has had for three years, he works as a senior principle engineer;

although, he still does not have a degree in engineering.

I asked Roz if Tim works with others who primarily have a bachelor's degree. She said no. She said that, in fact, many of Tim's colleagues have advanced degrees. So I then asked Roz how was it that Tim was able to do so much with one BS degree, and yet while she would soon have three lateral bachelor's degrees, why had these degrees not necessarily helped to advance her career? At the time, Roz was not aware of all the career possibilities that were available to her because no one had shown her the way.

By this point, you now know that I changed all that! Do you see what Tim had done in his career? He had built his base wide and strong and filled it with experience and knowledge. Tim had utilized the techniques that I have been speaking of. So I asked Roz why it was that she was not doing the same. Roz understood what I was saying and now utilizes these important techniques.

Build your base

Think *big*! Think *outside* the box! The next thing that I asked Roz is if her husband works with any nurses. Guess what? One week later, Roz returned to clinical and excitedly reported that yes, her husband works with many RNs. Imagine that: there are RNs working inside a medical device company who do *not* function in sales roles!

Hmm! Tim also had not even thought about it. He, too, had heard the word "nurse" and immediately envisioned his wife in a stereotypical nursing role. It was not until someone who was thinking outside the box orchestrated a conversation about alternate nursing possibilities that Roz gained more insight into the matter and realized how many career-changing opportunities there are out there.

Remember, it is about building your base wide and strong so that down the road, when you are laid off, you have a wide and strong base of knowledge and experience to pull from to help you land that next position. Really this is a biblical notion. Think about it: Build your house on a rock foundation, not sand, so that when the wind blows and the rains come, you can withstand the storm.

Online search

What? You are not aware of the wonderful opportunities within nursing? Is it because no one ever showed you what you could do or how to get there? Well, if that is so, those days are now over. I am here to show you a different way. I am here to show you where to look to find gems of nursing opportunities.

After you have gained one to two years of experience, you should hop onto Indeed.com and start searching with the keywords listed below. Indeed.com is my favorite job search engine because it is simple and easy to use. Indeed.com pulls from various sites including CareerBuilder.com, Monster.com, etc.

Additionally, while you are working in an RN position, *look* and think about all the companies that you deal with in your professional life. Make a list of these companies as you work! Keep in mind medical equipment and supply companies such as Hill-Rom and Baxter, pharmaceutical companies such as Pfizer and Merck, and lab companies such as Quest and LabCorp, among others.

Then, on Indeed.com, you can type in the name of one of these companies and do a search for available positions. For example, in the "what" search bar, type in "Baxter and Nursing" to find all the positions available that you can apply for!

Job keywords

If you do not have a specific company in mind, try some of these nursing positions as your keyword search instead.

- Advanced Practice Nurse
- Auditor Nurse
- Boards of Nursing
- Case Manager Nurse
- Clinical Documentation Nurse
- Clinical Educator
- Clinical Nurse Leader
- Clinical Nurse Specialist
- Corporate Nurse
- Correctional Nurse
- Dialysis Nurse
- Employee Health Nurse
- Executive Nurse
- FDA & Nursing
- Government/Governmental Nurse
- Health Management Nurse
- Home Care Nurse
- Home Health Nurse
- Home Infusion Nurse
- Hospice Nursing
- Industrial Health Nurse
- Informational Technology Nursing
- Insurance Nurse
- Joint Commission Nurse

- Kelly Healthcare Service Nurse
- Lab/Diagnostic Nurse (Sales/Marketing/Liaison)
- Legal Nurse Consultant
- LTC (long term care)
- Marketing and Nursing
- Materials Management Nurse
- Nurse Administrator
- Clinician
- Nurse Consultant
- Nurse Educator
- Nurse Executive
- Nurse Investigator
- Nurse Liaison
- Nurse Navigator
- Nurse Specialist
- Nursing Informatics
- Occupational Nurse
- Office Nurse
- Prison Nurse
- Public Health Nurse
- Quality Management Nurse
- Research Nurse
- Restorative Nurse
- Risk Manager Nurse
- Sales and Nursing
- Skilled Care Nursing
- SNF (skilled nursing facility)
- State Surveyor Nurse
- Telephonic Nurse
- Travel Nurse
- VA Nurse
- Wellness Nurse
- Worker's Compensation Nurse

HOLY COW! Do you see all these positions? Now go back and mix up these keywords... For instance, instead typing in "Home Health Nurse," try typing in "Home Healthcare Nurse." Or, instead of "Corporate Nurse," try "Corporate Executive Nurse." Or, instead of "Insurance Nurse," try "Nurse in Insurance." You get the idea! Also, look under "Sales" and/or "Marketing" and combine that with the keyword "Nurse." Why limit your possibilities?

What's the pay?

You need to know how much these prospective positions pay for two reasons. Firstly, you need to know if any of these possible positions are within your acceptable salary range, so you know if you are even able to consider making a career move or not. Secondly, you should know how much a position usually pays, so that you know if you are getting a fair offer or not when the time comes.

If you are not sure how much these positions pay, well, there is a website for that too! So, when you are ready to make a career change, be proactive and strategically position yourself to negotiate the salary that you deserve by using internet websites such as GlassDoor.com.

GlassDoor.com will afford you certain insights on a company, such as what the interview process may be like, what normal salary ranges are, etc. On GlassDoor.com you can even search open positions! GlassDoor.com is full of information, but I mainly use the website to search salary ranges, find the pros and cons of a company, find out what the interview process and timeline are like, etc.

It is important to note that the information you find on websites such as GlassDoor.com are opinions, so they may not be 100% spot-on. However, they offer you ballpark information, and if you do not utilize a website such as GlassDoor.com, you will not even have a ballpark estimation to reference. You need to know what a normal salary is before you can accept one, right? *This* is how to find out what the normal salary range for a certain position is!

> "When you undervalue who you are, the world will undervalue what you do and vice versa."
>
> -- Suze Orman

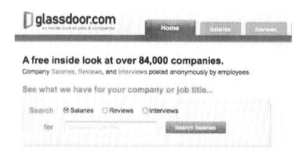

Referral networks

Next, have you thought about joining a referral network? Most people are hired because they are a referral from another person. Think about it. You hear about a job opening from someone. You ask the person if he or she can mention your name to HR or the hiring manager, and the process goes from there.

The same type of referral process happens when you know someone whose company has a job opening and you think about one of your friends as a possible fit. In this case, the referral and initial contact are made through you.

In fact, most positions are filled through networking, yet many RNs do not network outside the hospital. *Crazy*! As a nurse, you talk with people who have other occupations *all* the time. Think about the network that you could build by talking to *your patients* and their family members!

Friendliness pays

I was working as an RN in the L&D unit at a suburban hospital just outside the Chicago city limits. A woman and her husband came into the OB triage after being in a minor fender-bender. This was a precaution to monitor the mother for any potential contractions, as well as to assess the fetal well-being of the unborn child. As always, I was inclusive in my conversation with them and asked both of them what line of work they were in.

The wife informed me that she was a school principal, and her husband informed me that he was in my line of work. Joking with them both, I asked the woman if she planned to be the school principal of the school that their soon-to-be child would eventually attend, and I asked the man if he was a nurse who planned to become the school nurse at the same school. They both laughed. Then, the husband went on to say that he was in the healthcare industry.

Now, I could have stopped there, but I was inquisitive. So, I simply asked the husband what line of healthcare he was in. It turns out that he worked at a pharmaceutical company – the largest pharmaceutical company in the world!

Hmm, after hearing this information, I had to go on... I informed the man and his wife that I was trying to get into that line of work. He asked me a few questions, and guess what? I got an interview lined up from there! It turns out that this man knew a hiring manager who was looking for someone with a background in healthcare, which I had! No, I had never officially done sales before, but after three more interviews, I was hired.

I stayed at that company for eight years. Networking. It is very powerful.

More about Roz

Remember Roz? Well, on the day that her clinical group met for the last time, I took Roz and the group to meet and interact with several of the hospital's higher-ups who were also RNs. Roz and the group met the hospital's director of risk management, the chief cursing officer and the executive vice president. And because of the conversations that Roz had with these executives, a light bulb finally went off for her.

During her conversations with these prominently positioned RNs, Roz learned that there were more opportunities within nursing than she had previously thought. For example, the director of risk management had spoken to Roz about the attorney interactions that the position afforded her. This intrigued Roz.

Roz now realized how valuable her previous degrees could be in helping her build a bright future for her career as an RN. Roz had heard from me and was now hearing from others how many nursing possibilities lie ahead of her. If Roz frames her experience and education correctly on her resume (meaning that she properly emphasizes her knowledge, and personal or career growth), she can combine that with her two previous bachelor's degrees to build a very bright future, indeed!

Online networks

Now that you are beginning to see all the possibilities that are available for nurses these days, how will you go about networking? Again, look at the example of Roz and her husband Tim. Tim works at a large medical-device company and can easily help Roz network, even if he only helps her find internships, mentorships, or opportunities to shadow someone on the job. Thus, the question becomes, who can help you network?

Well, you have a professional networking website at your fingertips! LinkedIn.com can help you make networking contacts. This is an amazing site! It is strange to me that the majority of RNs are not familiar with LinkedIn.com. However, if I try to analyze why this is, I realize that it may be due to the fact that the basics of networking are simply not taught in nursing school!

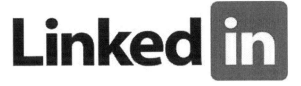

Now that you understand the value of networking and are being taught about the brilliance of a networking website, such as LinkedIn, I *strongly* suggest that you get onto LinkedIn.com and set up a basic account, which is free. This way, you can network with groups of RNs, seek out recruiters and network across the various business channels which utilize nurses.

By the way, nurses do not need to limit themselves on LinkedIn to networking with only other nurses and hospitals! Think about it. Nursing is a wonderful profession, and nursing opportunities are endless if you think about the bigger picture. So, build your network wide and strong, so that when you need it, it is there.

LinkedIn

Let me show you a few key points:

Once you have an active LinkedIn.com account, go to the top left tab titled "Contacts." From there, choose "Network Statistics" in the dropdown.

- Connections
- Imported Contacts
- Profile Organizer
- Network Statistics
- Add Connections
- Remove Connections

Look at these numbers! This member is connected with a whopping 147 people, which leads to more than 60,000 possible connections that are just one more contact-person away! Think about that!

LinkedIn.com also shows you area-specific growth, as well as industry-specific growth! Huge!

Here, you see statistics about your network, including how many users you can reach through your connections. Your network grows every time you add a connection, so — **invite connections now.**

Your Network of Trusted Professionals

You are at the center of your network. Your connections can introduce you to 4,760,500+ professionals — here's how your network breaks down:	
Your Connections Your trusted friends and colleagues	147
Two degrees away Friends of friends; each connected to one of your connections	60,200+
Three degrees away Reach these users through a friend and one of their friends	4,700,100+
Total users you can contact through an Introduction	4,760,500+

7,051 new people in your network since April 15

The LinkedIn Network

The total of all LinkedIn users, who can be contacted directly through InMail. **150,000,000+**

Total users you can contact directly — **try a search now!**

More About Your Network

REGIONAL ACCESS

Top locations in your network:

1. Greater New York City Area 7%

2. Greater Chicago Area 4%

3. San Francisco Bay Area 2%

4. New Delhi Area, India 2%

5. Greater Boston Area 2%

 Your region: Chattanooga, Tennessee Area

Your connections are in 36 locations but your network gives you access to **895 additional locations**, including:

Greater Atlanta Area
Greater Philadelphia Area
Greater Boston Area

Fastest growing locations in your network:

- Greater Chicago Area
- Dallas/Fort Worth Area
- Greater New York City Area

INDUSTRY ACCESS
Top industries in your network:

1. Human Resources   11%   ▬▬▬▬▬▬▬

2. Staffing and Recruiting   10%   ▬▬▬▬▬▬

3. Hospital & Health Care   9%   ▬▬▬▬▬

4. Pharmaceuticals   9%   ▬▬▬▬▬▬

5. Information Technology & Services 8%   ▬▬▬▬▬▬

 Your industry: Hospital & Health Care

Your connections are in 50 industries but your network gives you access to **148 additional industries**, including:

1. Telecommunications
2. Accounting
3. Construction
Fastest growing industries in your network:

• Information Technology and Services
• Financial Services
• Computer Software

I strongly encourage you to look at the "Groups" tab at the top. See? There are *so* many different nursing groups that await you! And guess what? Each group mentions more available positions, as well! Welcome to the endless list of potential career moves that nursing affords you!

So, revisit the above list of possible nursing positions that I have compiled for you, and ... think *big*! Think *really* big!

Different approach

In order to succeed – as I've said before – you must build your *knowledge*, take *action,* and overcome your *fear*. You must take the knowledge that I have given you – how to approach nursing from a critical (and crucial) business perspective – and combine that with action to land your dream job!

In this chapter, I hope that I have taught you to look at job opportunities in a different light and to think outside the box when it comes to finding your dream nursing position. My goals in this chapter were to show you how the nursing industry is a business similar to anything else and to illustrate ways in which you can network and find business opportunities.

In the next chapter, we will explore the pros and cons of pursuing graduate and post-graduate degrees as they pertain to nursing.

Chapter 10:

Beyond a Bachelor's Degree

If you decide that you want to go on to pursue a master's degree, I would encourage you to continue to think big. Time and time again, I see nurses who have been taught that they *need* a clinical or educational master's degree in order to obtain a higher rate of compensation. However, that is not what I have experienced, nor do I see this as a requirement when I perform numerous job searches on Indeed.com.

If you want to stay within the hospital or educational realm of nursing, then yes, a master's degree or even a post-master's degree will be in your future. However, nursing fields that exist outside a hospital setting, such as that of business and nursing, have proved that nurses in these settings need only experience and a bachelor's degree to receive competitive financial compensation.

Post-bachelor degree jobs

When I was starting out in nursing, I was told that there are two nursing fields that require a post-bachelor's degree: advanced clinical nursing and nursing education. Period. Thus, I chose to go

Carmen Kosicek, RN, MSN

the clinical route, and I obtained my MSN as a Nurse-Midwife. Because I have an MSN, I am able to teach at some colleges and universities. However, you should keep in mind that most universities only hire a limited number of full-time instructors who only have an MSN degree, so if you really, really, *really* want to teach at this level, you should pursue a doctoral degree, such as a DNP, EDD, PhD, etc.

Clinical roles are quickly changing in the current economic environment, and soon they will require a nurse to have a PhD or other doctoral degree. The downside to these evolving requirements is that they call for *a lot* of time and education, which can come with a hefty price tag. Not only that, but remember that having these pieces of paper does not necessarily guarantee a job, nor does it guarantee a higher-paid job.

Alternate paths

Let's think about it. Personally, I know *several* Advanced-Practice Nurses in many states who tell me that they can make more as a staff nurse than an Advanced-Practice nurse due to compensation that they receive from overtime, shift differentials and hospital-paid medical benefits. In contrast, working in their roles as Advanced-Practice Nurses comes with having to pay for malpractice protection and tail coverage on malpractice, as well as being limited in the number of available roles from which to choose. Sad but true.

You should also recall that educational debt usually follows you forever. This may be fine if you plan on pursuing a clinical or teaching role, which are *great* choices – don't get me wrong. However, I also want to present you with alternative nursing opportunities and roles for you to choose from, most of which simply require a bachelor's degree. By following any of these alternate paths, you will find more available positions to choose from, as well as a greater variety of the types of nursing positions that are offered. In addition, these alternate paths often simply pay more than the advanced clinical roles do, even though most nurses choose to go the latter route. Again, I am here to show you the world of opportunities that exist within nursing, but ultimately the choice is up to you.

If you do decide to pursue a post-bachelor's degree, do some research to unearth all the graduate and post-graduate degrees that are available to you. Find out if any of the available degrees or courses of study interest you, but also do your due diligence to see *if* the nursing positions that you are ultimately seeking even require or prefer these post-bachelor's degrees or not. There is a plethora of nursing positions outside the hospital that do not fit the stereotypical mold of what a nurse should be and that do not require advanced degrees – even though they may pay more than those stereotypical nursing positions which do require advanced education.

If you do choose to pursue graduate education, Google any of the topics below to see what may be of interest to you. Again, as you find topics that interest you, keep in mind which ones will help to advance your nursing career and which ones will not help to open doors in the field of nursing.

- Acute Care Nursing (NP/CNS)
- Adult Nurse Practitioner
- Certified Nurse-Midwife
- Community/Public Health/Home Care Nursing

- Family Nurse Midwife
- Family Nurse Practitioner
- Master's of Science Dual Degree Program in Nursing and Business Administration (MS/MBA)
- Nursing Business & Health Systems
- Nursing Education
- Nursing Entrepreneurship
- Nursing Healthcare Policy
- Nursing Informatics
- Nursing Management/Executive Leadership
- Nursing Quality and Patient Safety
- Pediatric Nurse Midwife
- Pediatric Nurse Practitioner
- Psychiatric-Mental Health Nursing (NP/CNS)
- Occupational Health Nursing

I realize that this is not an exhaustive list of graduate nursing options, but I simply want to show you how many *options* are out there, should you want to go on. First though, I encourage you to think about what it is that you want to do in your long-term nursing career, and find out if more education or another piece of paper is needed. Education is not free; it takes not only a financial commitment but a time commitment, as well. So, do your due diligence first to see what is truly needed to help you land your dream job.

> "Careful who you get advice from.
>
> I get advice from people who are where I want to be."
>
> – Robert Kiyosaki

Lucrative areas

Examples of lucrative areas of nursing that may not require a post-bachelor's degree? One example that first comes to mind is the pharmaceutical arena. This first pops into my mind because of my background. But you should know that, no, working for a pharmaceutical company does not always mean being involved in sales! Additional examples of lucrative areas of nursing that do not necessarily require education past a BS degree are insurance, research, biotechnology, and medical device, among others.

Now, go back to the list that I suggested on Indeed.com and look up prospective nursing positions that interest you. Next, look at the salary range of each position, which is located on the left-hand side of the page. Make sure to click on a few positions to see what level of education they require.

Don't forget that in terms of compensation, companies outside the stereotypical realm of nursing often offer better benefits than their traditional counterparts. This could mean better offerings in regard to healthcare reimbursement, prescription drug coverage, vacation time, 401(k) matching, etc. Dare to be different

I agree that your learning, or anyone's learning for that matter, should never stop. However, I hope that I have shown you that there are many ways to learn and many things to learn about. In this chapter, I have shown you alternative nursing paths to pursue that do not necessarily require graduate or post-graduate degrees but do offer competitive compensation and a unique working environment. In the next chapter, I will show you how to get noticed in the world of nursing and beyond.

Chapter 11:

Now What?

Sadly, most nurses and nursing students have on a set of blinders, which keeps them from seeing *all* the career options available to them. Fortunately, this book is designed to take the blinders off and show you the multitude of multi-faceted opportunities that is available for nurses! With this detailed guide, you are ready to embark on your *personal* nursing journey and succeed in this amazing career field.

Your future is limitless should you choose to think *big* and think outside the box in regard to the stereotypical nursing roles, which, in the past, have been presented to you as the only viable options for nurses.

Your resume

Now that you are ready to think differently and pursue different roles in your nursing career, you need to frame your experience appropriately. Yes, it is time to create your resume – and it needs to appeal to employers outside the traditional realms of nursing. Job competition is stiff, and in order to even be considered alongside other applicants and get past the first cut, your resume needs to entice and intrigue employers or managers who are not located in clinical settings. This means that your resume should stand out to nurse managers and businessmen alike.

The most important thing for you to do on your resume is highlight and emphasize your *results* at previous jobs. Do not merely state what your responsibilities were, and be sure not to simply state the obvious. Instead, share your success stories with prospective employers, whether these success stories are from Hospital ABC or the Pizza Palace.

For example, if you have been a bartender in the past, do not write on your resume that your skills include mixing drinks. Remember, do not state the obvious. Instead, on your resume, feature the hectic environment and the wide array of demanding people that you have successfully managed during your time as a bartender.

Show the growth!

Also, it is crucial for you to *show the growth* on your resume! By this I mean that you should show how you have grown within your previous job positions. One especially impactful way to demonstrate growth is to depict a percentage of growth through fiscal numbers. After all, even a hospital is a business, so share the numbers with them – that's what they need to see!

When trying to determine additional details that demonstrate growth at a previous company, you should ask yourself: Did you implement a new system that your employer and colleagues now use? Did you get a raise or a promotion? These details also show your growth at a company.

Remember, the *business* person or HR manager who first reads your resume will probably not understand nursing jargon as much as they understand *results*! So, show the growth!

In order to succeed, you must build your *knowledge*, take *action,* and overcome your *fear*. You must take the knowledge that I have given you – how to stand out in a sea of nursing applicants – and combine that with action to land your dream job!

A new perspective

I hope that by reading this guide, you have found yourself on an insightful and inspiring journey, one that will help you successfully traverse your nursing career in the years to come.

This may have been the first time that a nurse has been this transparent, honest and open with you! Thank you for being open to seeing that my thoughts and ideas are not far-fetched. Rather, the concepts that I have shared with you are realistic in the sense that they are integrated and supported by professionals outside the traditional realms of nursing.

I have been a nursing professor in a collegiate setting for more than seven years, yet I have taught throughout my entire healthcare career. You see, I *love* teaching others! And two of the main reasons that I teach are to stay current and to stay sharp.

I have taught a spectrum of people, from students to physicians. I have taught in colleges and to the number-one pharmaceutical-sales company in the world. I have taught techniques to laboring mothers to assist them in labor, and I have taught maximum security prisoners how to "hork" down charcoal. I love to teach!

In addition, my students always sing a familiar tune and say to me, "I have never heard it explained this way before," or "I understand it now," or "You are so different." I take these as the finest compliments because I strive to be different and shed new light on things! Throughout my entire life, I have never thought of myself as "normal." After all, *what is normal*?

Beyond 2012

My teaching style, as well as my life and nursing career, are not *normal.* My aim has always been to take something as complex as nursing and break it down for my audience. As I have done in this book, I strive to explain complex issues through stories and analogies, piece by piece, so that you will not only understand but *remember* what you have learned.

In turn, I want you to be able to implement the concepts and advice that I have shared, so that it positively impacts your life. In this sense, this clearly has not been a *normal* learning experience – it has been an educational opportunity!

Through sharing relatable and educational "stories," my goal is to get you to remember what you have been taught… In the long run, people do not remember concepts by memorizing facts and figures; instead, people remember stories. This is why I have filled this book with stories: to teach you in a way that you will remember.

Again, I am not a "normal" nursing teacher. Typically, a "normal" nursing teacher is more of a nurse than a teacher. Although I obviously have nursing skills, I find that my teaching style and content are influenced and inspired by many people, including those outside the direct field of nursing.

For instance, I am married to a Mastered-Prepared teacher who has home-schooled our two children, who are now teens. Thus, I have been greatly influenced on a daily basis by my husband's teaching style. Additionally, you have likely caught on by now that my teaching style has also been greatly shaped by key opinion leaders in the fields of business and finance, since there has been a massive infusion of businesspeople in the healthcare arena in recent years.

All of the concepts and techniques that I have learned from these influences have combined to change the way that I think, the way in which I perceive the future of nursing, the way in which I present, and the way in which I educate others.

More importantly, in 2012 and beyond, there has been a strong economic focus in the healthcare industry. Business, financial and legal aspects have converged with the world of nursing to create a melting pot of concerns surrounding healthcare and nursing.

Thus, in the 21st century and beyond, it is crucial for nurses and nursing students to think outside the traditional realms of nursing and learn alternative techniques and perspectives from someone like me – someone who offers a non-traditional approach to disseminating information, should you choose to learn and take action.

Embrace risk

Perhaps you are thinking that there are inherent risks in the concepts and techniques that I have discussed with you. To those people who are scared of risk, I ask you to consider this:

"Risk" (author unknown)

To laugh is to risk appearing the fool.

To weep is to risk appearing sentimental.

To reach out to others is to risk involvement.

To expose feelings is to risk exposing your true self.

To place your ideas, your dreams before a crowd is to risk their loss.

To love is to risk not being loved in return.

To live is to risk dying.

To hope is to risk despair.

To try is to risk failure.

But risks must be taken because the greatest hazard in life is to do nothing.

The person who risks nothing does nothing, has nothing, and is nothing.

They may avoid suffering and sorrow, but they cannot learn, feel, change, grow, love, live.

Chained by their attitudes, they are a slave; they forfeited their freedom.

> "There are two ways to face the future. One way is with apprehension; the other is with anticipation."
>
> -- Jim Rohn

I choose to face the future with anticipation! I sincerely encourage you to do that same!!

Build your base wide and build it strong. Remember to help others along the way. You will be an amazing nurse, no matter what path you choose! Indeed, I am the lucky one who was here to help lead and inspire you along the way!

> "You can't connect the dots looking forward; you can only connect them looking backward. So you have to trust that the dots will somehow connect in your future. You have to trust in something -- your gut, destiny, life, karma, whatever. This approach has never let me down, and it has made all the difference in my life."
>
> -- Steve Jobs

You can follow me at NursingCareerProfessionals.com or on Facebook at Facebook.com/NursingCareerProfessionals.

Personally contact me at info@NursingCareerProfessionals.com . One-on-one personal career coaching and speaking events are available, as well as information on how to fully protect your RN license.

ABOUT THE AUTHOR

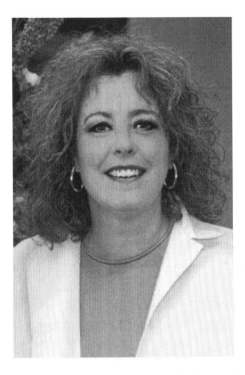

Carmen Kosicek has an extensive academic and professional background—in the fields of nursing and healthcare.

Carmen has helped hundreds of nurses and nursing students to envision a brighter nursing future filled with possibilities. With her love of business, she has assisted her nursing clients to increase their incomes by 20 percent or more within 18 months.

Contemporary, passionate and thought provoking, Carmen challenges nurses with support, encouragement and guidance to reach beyond their envisioned expectations. She guides them, with step-by-step techniques on how they can position themselves in the nursing field for continued career growth and success. Carmen explicitly presents a 21st Century proactive approach affording nurses the opportunity to protect their coveted RN license within today's vicious litigious arena—above and beyond traditional malpractice coverage.

Carmen's career began when she earned an associate of applied science degree in nuclear medicine from Triton College in River Grove, Ill., a bachelor of science in nursing from St. Joseph College of Nursing at the University of St. Francis in Joliet, Ill., and a master of science in nursing with a 4.0 GPA from the globally-recognized leader in nursing education, The Frances Payne Bolton School of Nursing at Case Western Reserve University in Cleveland, Ohio.

Carmen pursued her postgraduate education at one of the top 15 nurse-midwifery and nurse practitioner programs in the country, Frontier University in Hyden, Ky., where she obtained a certificate as an Advanced Practice Nurse in nurse-midwifery. Additional studies in healthcare economics and disease management led Carmen to a CMR certificate from the Certified Medical Representative Institute in Richmond, Va.

Intrigued by the expanding field of healthcare economics, Carmen became a licensed health, life, and legal agent with the Illinois Division of Insurance. She has continued fueling her commitment to lifelong learning with courses at The Rich Dad Education Co. and Tigrent Learning.

Carmen also has gained a wide array of practical, firsthand

experience in nursing and business. Many of her inspirational insights come from the broad and strong knowledge base she built throughout her healthcare career.

Carmen started her healthcare career as a certified nuclear medicine technologist and went on to land her first BSN-RN position straight out of nursing school in women's health—labor and delivery. She then became an OB Nurse Manager and finished her full time clinical nursing career as an Advanced Practice Nurse-Midwife.

The business world pulled Carmen into healthcare sales. Eight years with Pfizer Inc., once the world's largest pharmaceutical company, gave Carmen solid, foundational knowledge of the field.

Keeping active in nursing via Maxim Healthcare Services, the largest privately held healthcare staffing company in the nation, Carmen's healthcare experience expanded in the arenas of maximum security prison nursing, hospice nursing and community health nursing.

Then collegiate education and writing came calling. For eight years, Carmen has been a nursing adjunct professor in both ADN and BSN programs in the private and for-profit sectors. In 2012, she became a director of development in Nursing & Health Professions for Corinthian Colleges Inc., one of the largest post-secondary education companies in North America. In July 2012, she decided to share and publish her knowledge.

Nurses, Jobs and Money is her first book—it's a must-read for every nurse and everyone who is one and/or wants to become one!

Carmen, her husband of 22 years, and their two children reside just outside of Chattanooga, Tenn., overlooking the Appalachian and Cumberland mountain ranges on Signal Mountain, Tenn.

To contact Carmen for one-on-one mentoring, to learn how to protect your RN license, or to book her for a speaking event at your college or post college venue, go to www.NursingCareerProfessionals.com or contact her at info@NursingCareerProfessionals.com .

"Finding a good mentor will help bring out the best in you when you don't necessarily see the qualities you possess. Talent cannot be taught which is why coaches are more valuable than players. Without good coaches, the importance of talent would be diminished

Many people who want to succeed start to move forward in their discipline, and in doing so, they outgrow the current group of people they spend most of their time with. At that point in their career, to succeed, they are faced with the prospect of changing over to something new or remaining with that same group. In order to move forward, they may need to change to a new group because sometimes when a person grows and moves forward, those in their current group may be resentful, possibly because they feel stuck and are not moving forward or do not have the motivation to move forward. I personally make it a practice to never spend time around negative people. If I find a negative person in my life, I move on quickly. I always say discard negativity from your life. The top people in any field are never negative. They don't have time for that."

-- John Lang

FIND OUT MORE

Carmen's vision is to continue to uplift nurses, as well as nursing students, to the complete spectrum that is obtainable within the RN realm. For further information on how to book Carmen for one-on-one career coaching, events at you school, your hospital or to learn how to fully protect your RN license, reach out to Carmen directly at info@NursingCareerProfessionals.com

Carmen empowers nurses on how to expand their careers, salaries and vision. Visit www.NursingCareerProfessionals.com to learn about the latest offerings that Carmen is personally giving to each and every RN and SRN.

Carmen welcomes groups of any size to invite her in for speaking engagements at colleges and/or post college venues. Her talks and events show RNs how they can advance into further and higher paid positions within nursing. Carmen additionally covers what every nurse of the 21st Century needs to fully protect her/his coveted RN license.

You can reach Carmen at info@NursingCareerProfessionals.com or www.nursingcareerprofessionals.com/ .

You can also join her professional network on LinkedIn and/or follow her on Facebook at

https://www.facebook.com/NursingCareerProfessionals .

Network with other nurses via Carmen!

16972021R00092

Made in the USA
Lexington, KY
20 August 2012